DR RANJ SINGH

SAVE MONEY

LOSE WEIGHT

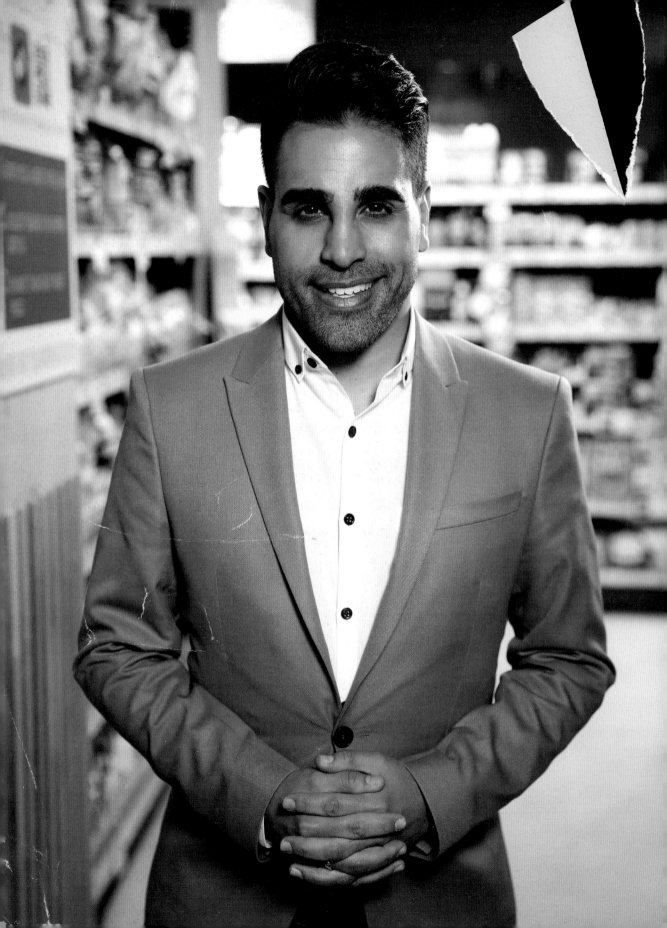

DR RANJ SINGH
SAVE MONEY LOSE WEIGHT

Spend less and reduce your waistline with my 28-day plan

Recipes by Georgina Davies

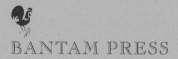

BANTAM PRESS

TRANSWORLD PUBLISHERS
61–63 Uxbridge Road, London W5 5SA
www.penguin.co.uk

Transworld is part of the Penguin Random House group of companies
whose addresses can be found at global.penguinrandomhouse.com

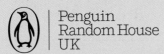

Penguin
Random House
UK

First published in Great Britain in 2019 by Bantam Press an imprint
of Transworld Publishers

This book is published to accompany the television series entitled
Save Money Lose Weight, first broadcast on ITV in 2019. *Save Money
Lose Weight* is produced by Twofour

Executive Producer: Rachel Innes-Lumsden
With thanks to Shirley Patton

A CIP catalogue record for this book is available from the British Library.

ISBN 9781787632486

Typeset in 9/12pt Gotham by Smith & Gilmour
Printed and bound in Italy by Printer Trento S.r.l

Text Consultant: Nicola Lafferty
Nutrition Consultant: Professor Jane Murphy
Editorial Director: Michelle Signore
Project Editor: Jo Roberts-Miller
Text Design and Art Direction: Smith & Gilmour
Food Photography: Jamie Orlando Smith
Food Stylist: Phil Mundy
Props Stylist: Olivia Wardle
Recipe Writer: Georgina Davies georginadaviesfood.com

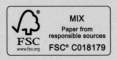

MIX
Paper from
responsible sources
FSC® C018179

13 5 7 9 10 8 6 4 2

CONTENTS

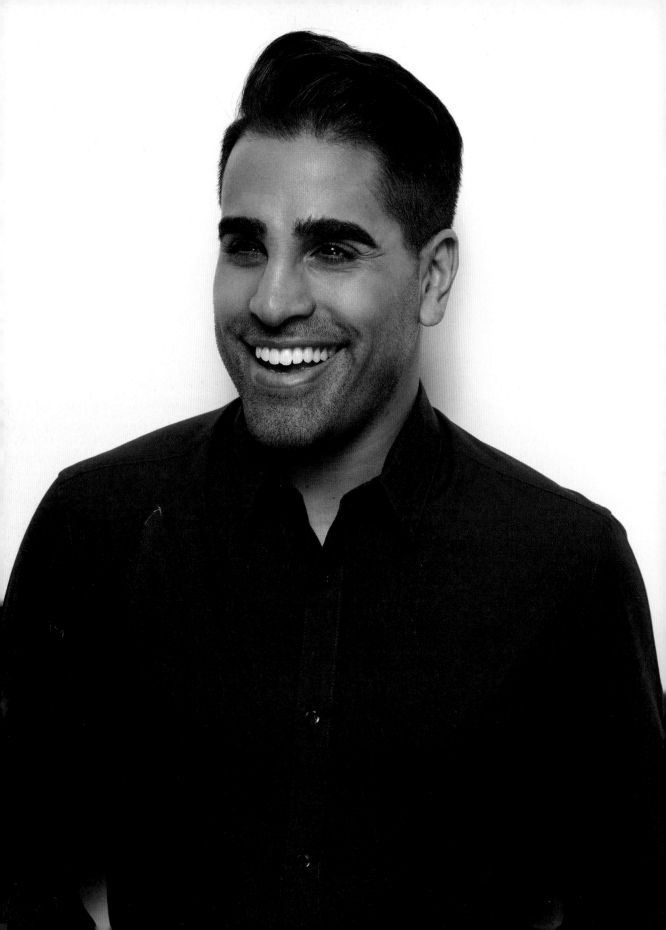

WELCOME

I've worked in the NHS for the last 15 years, and for most of that I've specialised in Paediatrics. During this time I've seen lots of children, families and adults struggling with weight-related issues. I've also seen how their lives can be transformed by making some very simple, affordable changes to their diets and lifestyles. It's shown me that my role is not just to cure physical ailments, but also to help people feel better physically and mentally – and taking control of your diet and weight can work wonders for your self-esteem and confidence.

I've also experienced this first-hand for myself and it's got me really fired up about healthier eating. I didn't have a very balanced diet growing up, which meant I was overweight as a kid and then carried some of those struggles through into adulthood. The reasons for this were complex; it was partly down to the environment I grew up in, partly because we didn't really understand healthier choices, and partly because those choices felt out of reach, either practically or financially. Trust me, I know just how hard it is to eat healthily, especially in a busy, working family!

I'm still constantly trying to maintain a healthier weight, sometimes with more success than at other times. I have a seriously sweet tooth and am always having to rein it in, and at the same time trying to motivate myself to do exercise. For me, it's not about being skinny, but being a comfortable, healthy size and feeling good about myself. Personal experience has shown me the confidence-boosting effects of losing weight, and I've learned that a bit of knowledge alongside some savvy shopping is all that it takes. That's exactly why I'm passionate about showing others how to do it, too.

Here in the UK we spend billions of pounds every year on trying to lose weight. It really can cost you a small fortune. The *Save Money Lose Weight* series has been on a mission to find which products are the most effective and which are worth spending your hard-earned cash on. In these programmes our plucky diet road testers have trialled the most up-to-date and popular diet books, plans and products. We've worked out how much each pound lost really costs in cash terms, and learned lots of amazing tips and tricks along the way. I've shared many of these with you in this book so some of the legwork has been done already. We show you it's possible to shed the pounds without spending a packet.

I've definitely put my money where my mouth is, too. The costly and sometimes traumatic lengths that some people will go to in order to lose weight fascinate me, which is why I've put myself in the hot seat and been the 'extreme diet guinea pig' on the series. I've tried some of the strangest diets on the market and some of them, such as the bone broth fast, I won't be trying again – and you don't need to either!

You see, I believe that healthier eating shouldn't feel like a punishment, because, if it does, you won't maintain it in the long term. 'Diet food' doesn't have to be boring, expensive, or feel any different from normal food. All it takes is a bit of thought and planning, which I've tried to do for you, so you can make healthy, low-cost, low-calorie choices for life. This book is packed with recipes that you and the rest of the family can enjoy together, so no more lonely diet meals for one. Also, I've made sure to include some treats and tipples, too, so you can enjoy yourself now and again! The less isolated you feel on your diet, the more likely you are to stick with it.

The same is true of exercise. It took me nearly 40 years to discover my love of dancing, and it is now my favourite way to stay in shape. Like healthy food, it doesn't have to be high cost. It is often free and the benefits aren't just physical – the mental and social benefits are massive. And the best part of it all: it doesn't feel like exercise!

None of this can be achieved if you don't aim for your goals. I've always believed in aiming as high as you can in life – it's certainly worked for me! I didn't start with a privileged life and I never believed I could become a doctor; I didn't think I was clever enough and my family weren't particularly well off. However, at a crucial point in life someone gave me some great advice; they said, 'Aim for the best you can be; even if you don't achieve it, you'll be in a better place than when you started.' I've used this advice again and again as my personal motivation whenever I've needed to make a big change, and I've never been disappointed. There is no such thing as all or nothing – it's always all or something.

I didn't think I would ever write a book either, but here I am. This book has one aim – to help you reach a healthier weight in an achievable, affordable and enjoyable way. It's not supposed to be a challenge or a chore, but a journey of learning, trying things out and finding what works for you. Follow some of the tips, advice and recipes, and even if you have a few slip-ups along the way, don't worry because you'll still be in a better position than when you started. By reading this you've already taken the first step!

Now let's keep going and get you to that healthier weight and lifestyle, and hopefully a happier you. I did it, and so can you!

Ranj X

THE SAVE MONEY MESSAGE

The ambition of *Save Money Lose Weight* is to interrogate and road test every product, gadget, gizmo and diet plan that is marketed towards losing weight. We'll put anything through its paces, from whichever diet book is topping the Amazon bestseller list to the hottest diet food or fasting craze, the latest weight-loss treatment and off-the-shelf diet foods. We leave no stone unturned! Everything goes through the same *Save Money Lose Weight* filter; will it help me lose weight and is it worth the money? Our main focus is always to keep as many of your pennies in your purse as possible. We really are very geeky about it and get a genuine kick out of reading food labels and comparing products and costs for you. If we can find a saving that no one else has spotted then we are over the moon!

It's not just about saving you money at all costs, though. We always want the quality of the lower price options we recommend to be on a par with your first-choice foods. We look at lots of products that are marketed towards dieters, such as low-calorie and 'light' foods, and compare these to the regular, best-selling versions. Sometimes the 'light' versions can be a great switch when you are on a diet, but occasionally they make no real calorie saving and actually cost more money. The answer is to read the labels carefully to find out which are worth switching. These simple swaps can mean massive savings for your food bill, and with a few tweaks to portion sizes you can still control your calories in exactly the same way.

Own brands and low-cost supermarkets feature a lot in our tests and comparisons. We trawl the aisles looking for good, low-cost and low-calorie alternatives. Not all of the product information for these foods is available online, so we get down there and check out the prices for ourselves, and for you, too, of course.

While savings are very important to us, we also know that life is busy and that many of us have jobs, families and responsibilities. Sometimes we all need to pick up a quick meal or snack on the run to keep our diet plans on track. Eating freshly cooked food every day is the best option but we understand that emergencies happen. We still want you to have the best that you can have for your budget, so we always road test the ready meals on the TV series, too.

I believe that you can be healthy without the need to be wealthy. There is actually very little evidence that one weight-loss plan is better than any other – it is sticking to the plan that counts and maintaining a healthy lifestyle thereafter. Spending lots of money on expensive foods and products just isn't necessary. Reasonably priced ingredients that you can buy in normal supermarkets will work just as well.

The market is flooded with advice on how to lose weight quickly, but not all of these plans and products take your long-term health into account or the fact that you may be on a tight budget. If you are going to spend your hard-earned cash on these products, then I want you to understand what they will and won't do for you. Just as we do in the series, I want to help you make informed decisions about what to spend your money on (see How Diets Work: The Facts Behind the Latest Fads overleaf).

One minute we are being told to cut carbs, then we are downing protein shakes or cutting out dairy and ditching sugar, too! Don't get me wrong, I know from my own experience that it can give you a brilliant boost to hop on the scales and see that you have made quick progress. It does wonders for your motivation when your clothes feel looser and you feel energised, too. In a way, the kind of diet you choose to start off with is less important than the fact that you are getting started (as long as it is healthy!). You are already on your way to a much healthier lifestyle – well done.

However, the best eating plan is one that is well balanced and that you can stick to long term, but before you start any diet it's important to understand what the plan really means for you and your health.

N.B. Speak to a healthcare professional if you have any concerns or have a long-term health issue that would be affected by a diet plan.

HOW DIETS WORK: THE FACTS BEHIND THE LATEST FADS

HIGH-PROTEIN/HIGH-FAT/ LOW-CARB DIETS

These have been popular diets for many years. Recently, plans called 'keto' have been grabbing the headlines. Sometimes these diets are used to treat medical conditions. Generally speaking, these plans all advocate low-carb eating, with generous portions of protein and fat on the menu. With keto plans, in particular, the body is described as going into 'ketosis'.

What is ketosis I hear you ask? We normally depend on glucose as our primary form of energy. If we are on a low-carb, high-fat diet, there is not enough glucose available to meet our energy demands and the body begins to break down fat stores instead. Ketosis describes the process by which the body converts these fat stores into energy, releasing ketones in the process. As one of our diet road testers discovered, you can test your levels of ketosis by using a special stick to test your urine – the colour of the stick will tell you if you are in a state of ketosis.

Eating lots of butter, eggs and bacon may feel like a really brilliant, if slightly bonkers, way to lose weight, but there's no such thing as a free lunch and eating foods that are high in saturated fats can increase your cholesterol levels. The total elimination of other food groups can also lead to nutrient deficiencies. Headaches, constipation, bad breath and short-term fatigue are some of the less fun side effects that people can experience. For most healthy people, these diets aren't harmful as a way to kickstart weight loss but, in my view, should be used for a short time only.

GUT HEALTH DIETS

In the series we dedicated an entire episode to gut health and it was really fascinating to understand what a big impact it can have on our general wellbeing. Gut health diets recommend lots of whole grains, fermented foods, cutting out sugar and giving up alcohol. Plenty of vegetables and fruit are also key.

The gut is home to the microbiome, which is made up of microbes that do some pretty important work, including taking the bits of food that our bodies can't digest, e.g. in fibre, and turning them into a small amount of additional nutrients, e.g. B vitamins and vitamin K, that the body can absorb as well as gases. These can influence our mood, appetite and general health.

The foods recommended on these diets claim to help your microbiome to thrive, promoting weight loss. These healthy foods are highly likely to improve your weight loss chances, but whether or not they improve your gut health could be very specific to you, as no two guts are the same. In cost terms, these plans can stretch the food budget considerably.

MEAL REPLACEMENT PLANS

Meal replacement plans work by replacing some or all of your meals with nutritionally balanced, calorie-controlled powdered shakes, soups, meals or bars. On the series we have road tested many of the most popular products. Some plans involve gradually reintroducing normal food and many offer additional support in the form of group meetings and online communities.

Recent studies advocate the use of these plans to kickstart rapid weight loss. In fact, there is now good evidence that very low-calorie meal replacement plans can reverse type 2 diabetes. It was believed that you might put the weight back on more quickly if you lost it using products like these, but that isn't the case. If your health is at risk from diabetes or other serious weight-related conditions, then some of these plans may be a good option for you to start off, before turning your attention to finding a healthy and sustainable way to manage your diet for the future.

These plans are easy to follow and the limited nature of the food on offer can help your to steer clear of the temptations that often trip up our diet plans in the early stages. Even if small weight loss is achieved, it can bring both immediate and lasting health benefits, and, in cost terms, the products can be very affordable. As ever, making the switch from the shakes and bars back to a healthier diet is the challenge. The support that some of the group meetings offer can help keep those early diet plans on track, but a monthly subscription could cost anything up to £25, on top of the product costs.

A MEDITERRANEAN DIET

There isn't one definitive Mediterranean diet but, generally speaking, it incorporates the dietary and lifestyle habits of people in countries bordering the Mediterranean. It is rich in fresh vegetables, fruits, nuts, seeds, beans, lean meats, poultry and fish, allowing for the generous use of olive oil and even moderate amounts of red wine. This diet pattern emphasises a wide variety of whole foods and healthy fats, while limiting unhealthy saturated and trans fats, refined foods and sweets.

Eating plenty of fruit, vegetables and oily fish is great. Keeping a limit on red meat is also good. However, lots of fresh food and a lot of olive oil might stretch your grocery budget a bit further than usual.

PALEO

The paleo diet only allows foods that can be hunted, gathered or fished (if you have the time!). It is based on the theory that our bodies are designed to eat like our caveman ancestors and that they're not designed to digest processed foods, which are the basis of our modern diets. Dairy, grain, pulses, starches, alcohol, processed foods, sugars and sugar substitutes are no-nos.

You may feel better overall and lose some inches around the waist as you cut out empty calories from processed foods. With the elimination of grains, this diet can be lower in carbohydrates as well. You may feel a bit deprived as you cut out junk and, because this diet is restrictive and eliminates many food groups, you may need to supplement certain vitamins or minerals. Also, this diet is far from the mainstream lifestyle many people currently follow, so it may be challenging to eat like a caveman long term. We also found that this was an expensive diet.

VEGAN

If you feel that you are ready for a complete and utter diet overhaul, a vegan diet contains no animal products. This means no milk, no chocolate (unless it is vegan chocolate, which is expensive), no honey and definitely no burgers! Instead, you focus on grains, fruits, vegetables, pulses, nuts and vegetable oils. A plant-based diet would be high in anti-oxidants and will be packed with hunger-satiating fibre. Anti-oxidants may prevent or delay some types of cell damage and are found in many foods, including fruits and vegetables. Other benefits of the diet include being relatively low in salt and saturated fat.

Statistically, the Body Mass Index (BMI – see page 23) of vegans and vegetarians is much lower than those of us who follow a typical western diet, but if a vegan diet is not well balanced and varied, you may find yourself lacking in essential nutrients (such as calcium, iron and vitamins B12 and D) and protein, which are essential for all of us and especially for people who exercise a lot.

A part-time vegan plan could be a good way to ease the transition, including lots of fruit and veg into your diet, while still benefiting from other sources. Shopping savvy for good deals on fruit and veg will help you to manage this diet without breaking the bank.

INTERMITTENT FASTING (IF)

Intermittent fasting is a pattern of eating that combines a set time for eating with an extended period of fasting or very low-calorie intake. In the 5:2 method, you stick to your normal calorie allowance for 5 days of the week then fast (only consuming 500–600 calories) for 2 days. In the 16:8 diet, however, there is an 8-hour feeding period, during which you can eat anything you want, followed by a 16-hour fast.

The idea is that when you fast, you reduce your exposure to fluctuations in hormones, such as insulin. Levels of insulin rise after you eat and, in a sense, help the body to store fat. If you eat and snack constantly throughout the day, any type of fasting would reduce your total calorie intake and, therefore, weight loss would naturally follow.

However, fasting can make you 'hangry' and there could be a temptation to binge eat when you are not fasting, which may make this plan tricky to stick to long term. If your own diet is generally healthy, this is an easy switch to try and shouldn't cost you more on groceries.

DIET CLUBS, GROUPS AND SUBSCRIPTIONS

There is scientific evidence to suggest that we have more success with our weight-loss plans (and indeed our exercise plans) when we are supported by other people. There are many well-known diet clubs and groups that offer detailed calorie-controlled diet plans. Some even have own-branded ready meals that you can buy from the supermarket, which means you don't have to cook. It is easy to tot up your calorific intake each day, which will help you lose weight. You can also attend weekly meetings for inspiration and encouragement. This will cost you £20–25 per month, on top of the food you will need to buy to follow the recipes or eat the ready meals.

These plans give the dieter a really clear structure to work within and the option of group and even personal support in some cases. Many provide recipes that the dieter can continue to use to sustain weight loss over the long term and they always come in on the more reasonably priced side during our road tests.

RAW FOOD DIETS

These plans involve eating raw fruits, vegetables, grains, nuts and seeds. Raw eggs and fish (in the form of uncooked sashimi), meat (carpaccio) and raw dairy products are also sometimes included in these diets. Raw food enthusiasts believe that cooking food destroys its nutrients and natural enzymes. Enzymes are required by your body to assist in the breaking down of food, so the raw food movement believes that you can maximise these nutrient benefits by eating raw.

In terms of flavour and texture, this plan is going to be a very big adjustment for most people. You will need to quit refined sugars, caffeine and alcohol, so this could be a bumpy ride for some. It is cooking food that kills harmful bacteria (salmonella, for example), which may occur in some foods, so great care must be taken. Eating out could be very tricky and expensive, too.

JUICE DIETS

Juice diets often promise very quick weight loss – as much as 7 pounds in 7 days in some cases, which is far in excess of the recommended NHS safe rate to shed the pounds. While eating more fruit and vegetables is a good thing, you do need to ensure that you are consuming the correct number of calories required each day and that you get all the necessary nutrients for your body to function properly, as the diet may not be nutritionally well balanced. The natural sugars in fruits will cause a sudden energy boost once they are consumed, but dieters can experience a major crash in energy levels afterwards. Giving up caffeine is also recommended by many of these diets, which may cause nasty headaches for some.

This type of diet is not sustainable over a long period, but juicing may be a good way to incorporate more fruit and veg into a balanced diet.

WEIGH – HEY!
If you have a small set of digital scales, keep them where you can reach them easily. People forget that you can put a pan or a bowl on the scales and then zero the scale. You can weigh rice, cereal, vegetables, chopped chicken, or whatever you are going to cook or eat, easily and quickly.

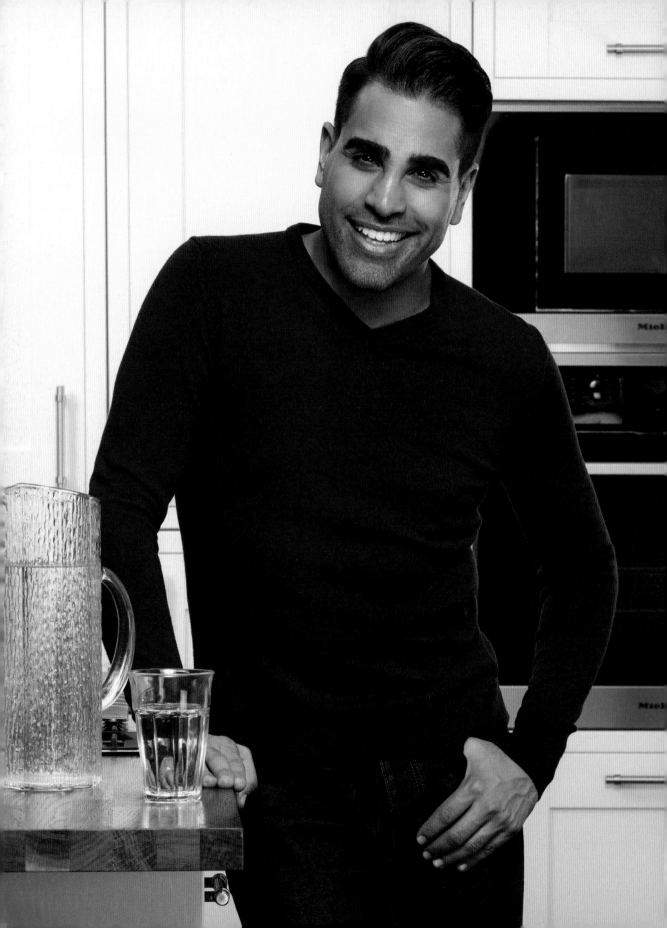

BEFORE YOU BEGIN

Change can be tough, especially when it comes to changing food habits that have been with you for years. You can always find a reason to avoid these difficult adjustments, and we are surrounded by temptations that trip us up along the way. In fact, calorie cutting and changing food habits are only a tiny part of what it takes to make lifestyle changes this big.

I have written a whole section on the techniques that I use when I need to shake myself up to get ready for big adjustments (see pages 19–22) but, for a start, our dieters in the series certainly benefited from getting mentally prepared. We made sure they talked about their goals with our team, and we got them to look back and question why certain diets hadn't worked for them in the past. We asked them to identify why it was so crucial for them to achieve success this time and we weighed them for the cameras and asked them to commit to sticking to their guns. By taking time to think things through before you start, you are much more likely to achieve success. And there are lots of ways for you to do this at home – you don't need the TV cameras!

Once you've thought about your personal motivation, assess your environment and see how you can make it more diet-friendly. Think about your home, office, or maybe even your car – where does the unhealthy eating happen and why? We've learned lots of tactics from our dieters to help you get prepared (see pages 21–22 to diet-proof your home). The methods we describe are all ways for you to plan for success, and there are lots of other tips and tricks in these pages that will help you to achieve your goal without breaking the bank. Saving you money is at the absolute heart of everything that we do on the series. You also need to take a good look at what you are eating, though, and my guide to calories and portion sizes will help you make better food choices straight away. Exercise is really important, as well, and it needn't cost you anything. My ideas for low- and no-cost exercise will get you off the sofa and moving in no time (see pages 44–47). Try it for the 28 days of our plan and you will feel the benefit.

You may have tried diets before that didn't work. Perhaps the food on your chosen plan was very limited, or the exercise required was impossible to fit in with a normal working and family life. The diet business is a multi-billion-pound industry and often it's about selling you 'the next big thing'. Every day there is a new headline about food in the newspapers – avoid dairy, quit sugar, eat more protein, ditch carbs! It is confusing and also very easy to think that the latest book, craze or product (however costly) could be the answer to your prayers. You might be motivated by trends and like trying something new each time – that's fine if it helps you to kickstart your weight loss but, in the long term, you need to find an eating plan that you can sustain for life.

I believe that eating the right foods in the correct portions and getting yourself moving more are the simplest solutions. The 28-day meal planners, low-cost recipes and savvy shopping lists in this book will not only guide you for those first four weeks but also forwards into a happy and healthy future.

GETTING STARTED – CHANGE YOUR MIND

In the *Save Money Lose Weight* series, our dieters have really good reasons to lose weight and yet they still can't seem to get started, even though their existing food habits have caused them all manner of problems. Some have health problems like type 2 diabetes and some are too breathless to play with their very young children. Others can't face the prospect of buying a dress even though their wedding day is just months away. Many of us have the most compelling reasons imaginable and still find ourselves unable to make the necessary changes.

In the NHS we use a technique called motivational interviewing to help people find the internal strength they need to change their behaviours. I used this method myself when I wasn't doing enough exercise, even though I was feeling very out of shape and tired. I really interrogated myself and I realised that one of the things that was stopping me was the fact that I couldn't stand the faff of getting my exercise gear together. As soon as I forced myself to leave it all packed by the front door the night before, I had no excuse to dodge it anymore!

Take your time and think about the questions opposite. Some people find it helpful to write their answers down to read again later. Maybe the same notebook could be used to log your progress and daily calorie counting, too?

ASK FOR HELP

There is lots of evidence to suggest that the support of others plays a massive part in the success of weight-loss plans. Our dieters weigh themselves at the start of the process and this weight is recorded, so that their progress at the end of a month can be revealed. Why not do this with a family member or a supportive friend, or start a healthy-eating gang? Speaking openly about your goals will make them feel more achievable and you will get lots of moral support and encouragement in return.

FIND YOUR MOTIVATION

➲ How is your current weight affecting your life right now?

➲ What has worked for you in the past?

➲ On a scale from 1–10, how ready are you to make changes to your diet?

➲ What are your hopes for the future, if you are able to become healthier?

➲ How do you feel about changing your eating or exercise behaviours?

➲ How would you like your health to be different?

➲ What do you think will happen if your weight doesn't change?

➲ What are the most important things to you? What impact does your weight have on those things?

➲ What help do you need to succeed?

➲ What are some practical things that you need to do to achieve your goal?

➲ What things stand in the way of you taking a first step (e.g. child care, transport, distance, cost, accessibility)? How can you overcome these things?

YOUR RELATIONSHIP WITH FOOD

It's also worth having a better understanding of your relationship with food. We all have one and it is different for everyone. My weaknesses are cake and chocolate, especially when I feel really tired. After a long hard day, do you reward yourself with a big bowl of ice cream? Do you eat when you feel in a low mood? Our series dieters admitted to eating both when they are happy and when they are feeling down. Food is consolation when we need cheering up and a reward when we want to celebrate.

Help yourself change these habits by trying new tactics to help you cope without relying on food in this way. When all I feel like doing is eating cake, I try to choose something richer in protein instead, like a wrap with lean turkey, salad and grated veg, or some slow-release carbs – food that will give me energy for longer. The recipes and tips in this book will help you to make these swaps cheaply and easily.

Plan some new strategies to replace the old habits:

➲ Swap the large chocolate bar for a long bath at the end of a tough day.

➲ Add up the money that you would have spent on all that ice cream and put it towards something special that you really want to buy.

➲ Make sure you get plenty of good-quality sleep – being tired will make you want to reach for sugary quick fixes.

STAY SOCIAL

I believe that food and eating should always feel like an enjoyable aspect of your life, even if you are watching the calories. The pleasure of sharing a meal is not something you should have to sacrifice because you are on a diet – you should never isolate yourself. Eating with others is really important. The delicious recipes in this book are perfect for sharing with friends and family without derailing your diet and, over time, you will get used to adapting all dishes to suit your needs, even when you are in a café or at friend's house.

If we feel really confident about our new healthy food choices, then we can continue to enjoy meals with others, without feeling pressured into eating exactly the same as everyone else. You can have less bread, have your salad without the dressing or serve yourself smaller portions generally – or simply get into the habit of not finishing everything on your plate! Your healthy-eating plans will be far more sustainable if you can continue to enjoy food socially. Above all, never feel self-conscious or guilty about saying 'No thank you' to well-meaning hosts or family members. I grew up in a house where food was love and saying no was hard, but if you explain in advance the very good reasons why you won't be having quite as much cheesecake as usual, trust me, they will understand.

If you take a bit of time to put these building blocks in place before you start your journey, it will be easier for you to stay focused and get yourself to that healthy weight. Think positive!

IDENTIFY YOUR TRIGGERS
Be aware of triggers that are likely to lead you to overeat. Are there certain times of the day when you are more likely to want to eat? Does it happen when you are at home alone or if you drive past a fast-food restaurant. Planning ahead may help you cope with these triggers. Use distractions to help control your eating and take your mind away from food. Replace one behaviour with another – maybe go for a walk instead.

GETTING STARTED – ADAPT YOUR HOME

We are very strict with our dieters on the series – they have to get rid of all their sneaky food stashes before they start their new eating plans. For some people that will mean emptying their drawer full of sweets and chocolate, for others it's ditching their savoury crackers and cheese. We even had a lady who joked that the bread bin called out to her as she walked past it! For one of our most successful dieters, the prospect of quitting her sugary fizzy drinks was incomprehensible – until she lost three stone on a healthy-eating plan that banned them. She doesn't miss them quite so much now! Don't get me wrong, though, I firmly believe that we all need treats so we have included recipes that will enable you to have some treats while still keeping your diet on track and without costing the earth (see pages 169–203).

DIET PROOF YOUR HOME

It's hard to change long-standing habits, but you'll give yourself the best possible chance if you prepare. Here are some practical tips to help you diet proof your home:

➲ Use smaller plates; it will help you to control portion sizes.

➲ Spring clean your fridge – your fresh healthy ingredients will look way more tempting if they aren't hidden behind the cranberry sauce from last Christmas.

➲ Make sure you have plenty of food storage boxes to hand. You will need these to carry low-cost healthy lunches and snacks when you are on the go. They'll come in handy for leftovers and for batch cooking, too. No need to buy new storage boxes, just recycle what you have. From yoghurt pots to sour cream containers and butter tubs, there are plenty of opportunities to wash, save and reuse the plastics pots that come your way.

➲ Hydration is really important so get yourself a water bottle and make it your mission to keep it topped up with no-cost tap water. We often think we are hungry when in fact we are dehydrated. Have a drink of water before you start eating and you will feel full more quickly. Also, drink a glass with your meal since that will make you feel fuller, too.

➲ Create a place for the healthy snacks and fruit that you want to eat – fill a bowl with them and have it visible on the side in the kitchen. This will help you avoid temptation and may also help your family make healthier decisions, too.

➲ For the snacks/drinks that you find hard to resist, why not try labelling them with the correct portion size and, while you are on the diet plan, include the amount of exercise needed to burn off that portion.

➲ Choose one of the many free online calorie calculators. These can be downloaded on to your computer or mobile phone and used for free. It's so easy to monitor your intake and it helps keep you on track.

⮑ We all have weekly family rituals when we eat treats, like a movie night or a calorific Sunday roast. Think about how you want to share these meals and experiences, without derailing your diet. See if you can sneak some lower calorie popcorn past the rest of the family on movie night. If they enjoy it, you could all make the switch! Or you could choose a lean meat, such as chicken, for your Sunday meal, which is usually cheaper than red meat, too. And don't roast all of the vegetables in oil – you could steam some instead.

⮑ Swap your glass of wine on weeknights for a no-alcohol alternative, and choose cheap, low-calorie options for your low-key treat at the weekend. We tested low-cost, low-sugar wines on the series, and you can reduce your calorie intake per glass quite easily, so it is possible to make swaps. BUT some of our dieters felt they made more unhealthy food choices when they had a few drinks, which doubled the damage. Alcohol contains 7 kcals per gram, which has almost the same calorific consequences as pure fat (9 kcals/g), so if you don't want to derail your diet, then cutting back on booze could be your best bet.

HERE ARE SOME REALLY PRACTICAL THINGS THAT I DO TO HELP WITH TEMPTATION

⮑ If your plate is looking a bit sparse, fill it up with vegetables.

⮑ If you're craving a mid-morning snack, go for a piece of fruit.

⮑ Try not to eat while doing something that can distract you, such as working, reading or watching TV. This can make you eat more, and you won't realise that you are full.

⮑ Pay more attention to what you're eating; make sure you chew each mouthful slowly and thoroughly.

⮑ Don't put large serving dishes full of food on the table, as you will be tempted to pile on the portions and the pounds.

⮑ Have a break after your meal before you have dessert. It takes time for your brain to recognise that your stomach is full. Wait about 15–20 minutes before deciding if you need that extra course.

UNDERSTANDING CALORIES

A calorie is a measurement of the amount of energy in a food item or drink. On food labels, the calorie content is often given in kilocalories (kcals), which is another word for what is commonly called a calorie, so 1,000 calories will be written as 1,000 kcals. As a rough guide, an average man needs about 2,500 kcals each day to maintain a healthy bodyweight. For an average woman, this figure is about 2,000 kcals. These numbers will vary depending on factors such as age, size (height and weight) and how much daily physical activity you take. However, as a rough guide, if you want to lose weight, it is important to eat fewer calories than this.

I am not recommending that you eat the foods in the Working Off the Calories Chart [overleaf], but it can be shocking, in a useful way, to realise just how much exercise it takes to burn off the calories we eat. Many people think nothing of tucking into a bag of crisps with their sandwich at lunch time, but these add-ons can have huge calorific consequences. Becoming familiar with the calorific cost of your food is the key to losing weight.

An important part of a healthy diet is balancing the energy you put into your body with the energy you use. If we take more exercise, we will use more energy. If you eat more calories than the body uses, you will store the excess as fat. If we continue to do this (and it doesn't need to be a lot more each day), over time we will gain weight.

WHAT IS YOUR BMI?

Body mass index, or BMI, is a measure of your body size. It combines your weight with your height. The results of a BMI measurement can give you a rough idea about whether you are the correct weight for your height. You can find a very simple **free BMI calculator** on the NHS website. By entering a few basic details, you can establish how many calories per day you need to eat to achieve safe and steady weight loss.

BMI is just a guide, though. While it can tell you if you're carrying too much weight, it can't tell you if you're carrying too much fat. It can't tell the difference between excess fat or muscle and bone. Very muscular adults and athletes may be classed as 'overweight' or 'obese', even though their body fat is low. Conversely, adults who lose muscle as they get older may fall into the 'healthy weight' range, even though they may be carrying excess fat.

WORKING OFF THE CALORIES

	KCALS	WALK OFF	RUN OFF
Quarter of a large pizza	449 KCALS	1hr 23 mins	43 mins
Chicken and bacon sandwich	445 KCALS	1hr 22 mins	42 mins
Dry-roasted peanuts (50g)	296 KCALS	54 mins	28 mins
Medium mocha coffee	290 KCALS	53 mins	28 mins
Blueberry muffin	265 KCALS	48 mins	25 mins
Standard chocolate bar	229 KCALS	42 mins	22 mins
Packet of crisps	171 KCALS	31 mins	16 mins
Sugary soft drink (330ml can)	138 KCALS	26 mins	13 mins

[Source: RSPH]

I'm a sugar fanatic who started young. As a child I remember regularly eating biscuits for breakfast. My parents were not neglectful, they just thought that 'fed is best'. The result is that I now have a ridiculously sweet tooth. I've had to swap the sugars I crave for artificial sweeteners to keep my calories down.

Small changes to your diet can have a huge impact on your health. To make these changes you need to understand calories. Learning to tot up how many calories you consume throughout the day will not only help your weight loss but it will also help you factor in some treats – and we cannot do without treats!

In general, to achieve weight loss most men should consume no more than 1,900 kcals per day and most women no more than 1,400 kcals per day. The recipes and meal planners in this book are all based on those figures. Most people will lose weight at a safe and steady 1–2 lbs per week by sticking to this daily calorie allowance. The recipes in this book are all calorie counted and you can follow my simple meal planners to make sure that you stay within the recommended daily allowance for your weight-loss targets (see pages 210–16).

Using a **free calorie-counting app** might be helpful. It may feel a little slow to begin with, as you will have to enter foods one at a time to assess their calorific content, but it will soon become second nature.

Think about the calorie content of the foods that you eat. What does 100 calories of chocolate buttons look like? How much pasta represents a 100-calorie portion? How does this compare to 100 calories' worth of cucumber or salad leaves? We have taken photos of various foods to help you visualise what 100 calories looks like (see overleaf). You need to know this if you want to lose weight. A quick look at these photos will give you an idea of roughly how many calories you are currently consuming on a daily basis. I am always surprised by the hidden calories in things like a teaspoon of butter. Knowing what 100 calories looks like will also help you keep on track when you are eating out and socialising.

Calories are a very important guide to how much food you should eat in a day, but it's how you put the right combinations of food together that will ensure you reach the right balance of essential vitamins and minerals for a healthy lifestyle.

WHAT 100 CALORIES LOOKS LIKE *overleaf*

½ avocado	144g peas	166g grapes
1 banana	2 small pears	15g walnuts
27.5g uncooked brown rice	357g cauliflower	1 tbsp butter
400g raspberries	27.5g uncooked chickpeas	322g green beans
130g new potatoes	19g chocolate buttons	4 heaped tsp white sugar
38g crusty bread	22g crackers	24g Cheddar
555g cherry tomatoes	56g cooked pasta	1kg cucumber
1 large egg	1 tbsp peanut butter	

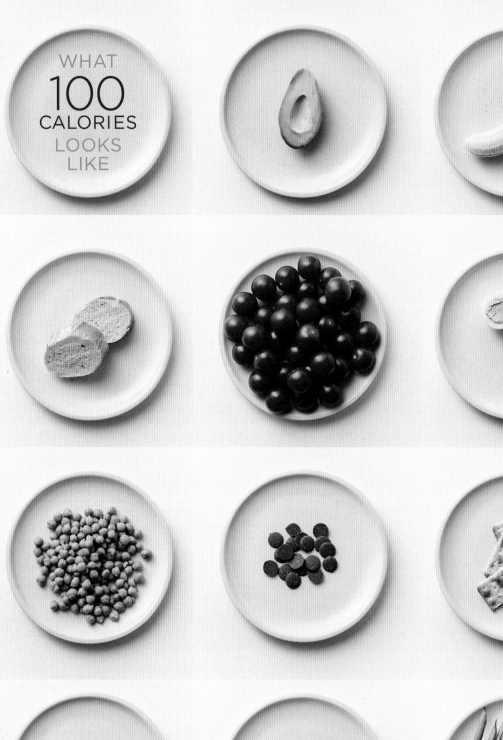

WHAT
100
CALORIES
LOOKS
LIKE

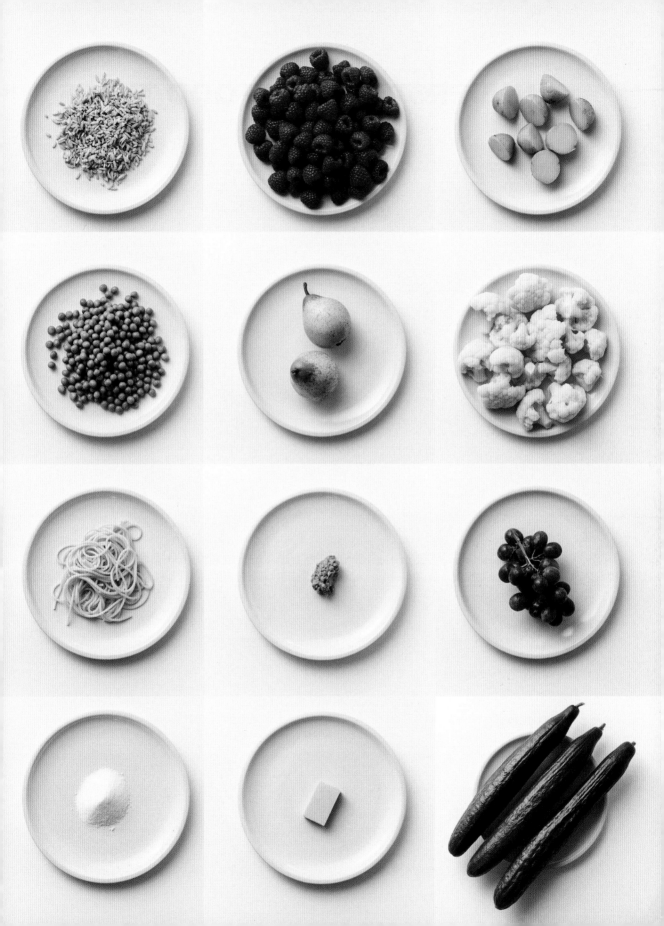

UNDERSTANDING FOOD TYPES

Getting to grips with the foods your body needs and how much of each food type you should eat is important. It can be hard to know where to begin, though. Before you get started, take notice of the food you currently eat every day, paying particular attention to the portion sizes. Here in the UK, the latest studies tell us that in general we eat too much saturated fat and not enough fruit and vegetables, and we are way down on what our fibre intake should be.

⮑ Only 31% of 19- to 64-year-olds, 32% of 65- to 74-year-olds and 8% of teenagers meet the 5-a-Day recommendation for fruits and veg.

⮑ The average fibre intake in adults is 19g per day, well below the recommended 30g.

⮑ The average saturated fat intake for adults (19- to 64-year-olds) represents 12.5% of their daily calorie intake, which is above the 11% recommended maximum.

The low-cost recipes in this book are all carefully worked out and balanced for you, so you will be off to a great start. We have also included four weekly meal planners (see page 210–16) to make the first 28 days of your healthy-eating plan as easy as possible.

WHAT MAKES A HEALTHY PLATE OF FOOD?

On Friday nights my parents did the grocery shopping, which meant that dinner on Friday was a feast, including homemade fish and chips and chocolate cake. Putting aside the hefty calorific content of that kind of meal for a moment (!), as a kid I also ate the same portion sizes as the adults – I had no idea what a balanced meal was. I certainly had never heard of saturated fats – it just wasn't something we knew about. As an adult, however, I have had body confidence issues and I know that the key to happiness for me is to stay at a healthy, happy weight. I do still struggle sometimes, but making sure that I eat the right portions of the right foods really helps.

⮑ **NON-STARCHY VEGETABLES on ½ of your plate** are vital because they have more fibre and fewer calories than starchy veg (like potatoes). They are nutrient-dense and can help lower blood sugar and cholesterol levels.

⮑ **STARCHY CARBS on ¼ of your plate** should be a fist-sized portion.

⮑ **PROTEIN on ¼ of your plate** should be the size of the palm of your hand. If you are cooking for children, please note that their portion of protein should be the size of *their* palm.

⮑ **FATS** on your plate, like butter, should be a portion no bigger than the size of your fingertip.

GUIDE TO A HEALTHY PLATE OF FOOD

½
NON-STARCHY VEGETABLES OR SALAD

¼
STARCHY CARBOHYDRATES

¼
PROTEIN

Ideally wholegrains like wholemeal bread, pasta, cereals, rice and potatoes (with skins for fibre). A quarter of a plate represents about 85g cooked rice, 110g cooked pasta or 3 egg-sized potatoes.

For example, spinach, cauliflower, avocado, mushrooms, pumpkin and lettuce.

For example, fish, eggs, soya, dairy, beans, pulses, chicken, turkey. A quarter of a plate represents about 100g fish or 90g meat.

PORTION SIZES

HAND
Non-starchy vegetables

PALM
Meats and other protein

FIST
Rice, pasta, breads and fruit

FINGERTIP
Fats (butter)

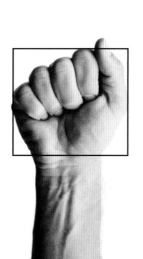
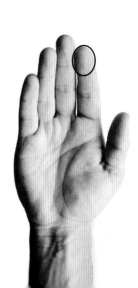

UNDERSTANDING FATS – THE GOOD, THE BAD AND THE UGLY

Fats get a bad rap but a small amount of fat is an essential part of a healthy, balanced diet. Fats are a source of essential fatty acids, which the body can't make itself and which help the body absorb vitamins A, D and E. All fats are also high in energy. The type of fat you consume won't make a difference to your calorie count: a gram of fat provides 9 kcals of energy, whether saturated or unsaturated (compared with 4 kcals for carbohydrate and protein). But your body handles them differently. If we eat too much of the wrong fats we can increase the risk of serious health conditions like heart disease, type 2 diabetes and some cancers.

We can't give up fat entirely, but we do need to educate ourselves about which fats to choose. As part of a healthy diet, we should try to cut down on foods and drinks that are high in saturated fats and trans fats, and replace them with unsaturated fat. Most foods usually contain a mixture of both types, so it's a bit of a minefield. To help you separate these fats into categories I have put them in colour-coded shopping baskets.

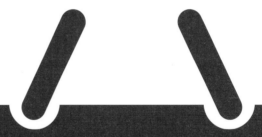

RED: SATURATED FATS = AVOID/LIMIT

Found in:
- ✗ Fatty meats
- ✗ Full-fat dairy products e.g. full-fat milk, hard cheeses, cream
- ✗ Butter, lard, ghee
- ✗ Palm oil and coconut oil
- ✗ Processed foods e.g. burgers, sausages, pies
- ✗ Some cakes, biscuits and pastries

THE BAD NEWS: Saturated fats are mostly found in animal products and can increase your blood cholesterol levels [they contain a type of cholesterol called LDL (bad) cholesterol]. A tip is to check the saturates content per 100g on food labels: 5g per 100g is a lot; less than 1.5g per 100g is a little.

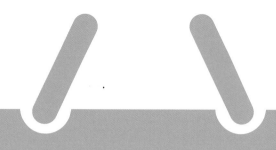

GREEN: UNSATURATED FATS = GO

Unsaturated fats help to maintain healthy cholesterol levels. There are two types of unsaturated fats:

1 **Monounsaturated fats** help maintain levels of good (HDL) cholesterol and decrease levels of the bad (LDL) cholesterol.

2 **Polyunsaturated fats** help to lower the bad (LDL) cholesterol and also provide us with essential fatty acids (which the body cannot make), such as omega-3 and omega-6.

MONOUNSATURATED FATS ARE FOUND IN:

- Avocados
- Olives and olive oil
- Rapeseed oil
- Almonds, cashews, hazelnuts, peanuts, pistachios and spreads made from these nuts

POLYUNSATURATED FATS ARE FOUND IN:

- Some vegetable oils and spreads e.g. corn and sesame
- Flaxseed, sesame and sunflower seeds
- Walnuts and pine nuts

Omega-3 polyunsaturated fats are mainly found in:

- Oily fish e.g. salmon, sardines, trout and mackerel
- Walnuts

There are some vegetable sources of omega-3 but they aren't thought to have the same benefits for heart health as the longer chain omega-3 found in oil-rich fish. If you don't eat fish, though, vegetarian sources of omega-3 include:

- Some vegetable oils and spreads e.g. rapeseed, linseed and soya
- Soya-based foods e.g. tofu

AVOID TRANS FATS

There are two types of trans fats; one is found at low levels in meat and dairy products, while artificially made trans fats, labelled as hydrogenated fats or oils, are found in some processed foods. Trans fats can also be found when vegetable oils are heated and reheated to fry foods at very high temperatures, so the most tempting of takeaways can be packed with these.

⮑ Vegetable oil can contain trans fats, so avoid those with 'hydrogenated fat' on the label. Helpfully most supermarkets have dropped these vegetable oils from their stores because of the health risks. Like saturated fat, trans fat can increase cholesterol, raising the risk of heart disease.

⮑ Here in the UK, thankfully, we don't eat a lot of trans fats. On average, we eat about half the recommended maximum BUT we eat a lot more saturated fats than we should! This means that when you are looking at the amount of fat in your diet, it's important to focus on reducing the amount of saturated fats.

WHAT ABOUT CHOLESTEROL?

In the past, we believed that eating foods containing cholesterol (e.g. eggs, liver, kidneys and shellfish) was the main source of cholesterol in the body. However, we now know that the amount of saturated fat in your diet has more of an effect on blood cholesterol. So, there is no need to avoid eggs, or the other foods, with respect to your cholesterol level, unless you have been advised to do so by a healthcare professional.

DON'T DESPAIR!

An important point to make is that there is no one food that is all bad. It is how you put foods together that makes them part of a healthy or unhealthy diet. Yes, butter is a saturated fat and ideally you should use unsaturated fats instead, but butter can be included in your diet if you do so sensibly. It all depends on what other saturated fats feature on your plate – if they come in the form of high-fat, refined sugary foods, you should be trying to cut back on them.

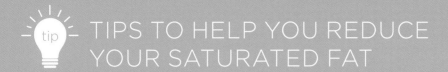

TIPS TO HELP YOU REDUCE YOUR SATURATED FAT

1 Swap butter, lard, ghee and coconut and palm oils for small amounts of monounsaturated and polyunsaturated fats, such as olive, rapeseed or sunflower oils and spreads. Most of the supermarket own-brand vegetable oils are rapeseed, which is one of the cheapest and healthiest oils you can buy.

2 Choose lean cuts of meat and make sure you trim off and discard any excess fat. It is also important to remove the skin from chicken and turkey. Turkey breast mince is a great swap for beef or lamb mince as it has far less fat.

3 Read food labels to help you make choices that are lower in saturated fat.

4 Grill, bake, steam, boil or poach your foods instead of frying them.

5 Make your own salad dressings using ingredients such as balsamic vinegar, lemon juice and herbs, with only a dash of olive oil.

6 Use semi-skimmed, 1% or skimmed milk, rather than using whole or condensed milk.

7 Instead of pouring oils straight from the bottle, use a homemade spray bottle (see page 64) or measure them out with a teaspoon.

8 Cottage cheese, ricotta and extra-light soft cheese are examples of lower fat cheese options. Remember that many cheeses are high in saturated fat so keep your portions small – matchbox sized. Opt for strongly flavoured varieties that will have a bigger impact on the flavour of your dish without needing to be a large portion. Also, make sure you grate the cheese so a little goes a long way.

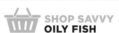

SHOP SAVVY
OILY FISH

Fish and shellfish are good sources of many vitamins and minerals. Oily fish, such as salmon, mackerel, herring, sardines and sprats, are all reasonably priced options. Oily fish are also particularly high in long-chain omega-3 fatty acids, which may help to keep your heart healthy. Some types of omega-3 cannot be made by the body so it is essential that we get them from our food.

UNDERSTANDING CARBOHYDRATES

Carbohydrates are an important nutrient, giving us around half of the energy we need every day. Most of us think of carbs as bread and pasta, but you can also find them in lot of other types of foods, too. Carbs are made up of three main components: fibre, starch and sugar. Fibre and starch are the good guys – these are the complex carbs – while sugar is a simple carb and one that you should seriously curb!

WHERE DO WE TRIP UP?

Many of us eat sugary cereal for breakfast, a sandwich on white bread for lunch and our evening meals will involve white pasta or potatoes. If we pile our plates too high with these foods then we will pile on the pounds, too. These carbs should be eaten in moderation or they will push up our sugar levels and, over weeks, months and years, increase our risk of heart disease and diabetes.

DITCH OR SWITCH THE CARBS

It's pretty easy to swap simple carbs for healthier complex carbs – switching from white bread to wholegrain is easy, ditching the white rice and using brown instead, or opting for wholewheat pasta. Lots of these 'brown' foods are more filling, release energy more efficiently, contain more fibre and extra vitamins and minerals, too. Also, why not eat your potatoes with their skins on? That's another easy way to get extra fibre into your diet! Remember – potatoes don't count as one of your five a day. They belong on the starchy/carb section of your dinner plate.

SHOP SAVVY
COMPLEX CARBS

Carbs that take longer to digest are better for you, making you feel fuller for longer and less likely to snack in between meals. This makes wholegrain foods a good choice, so stock up on sweet potatoes, wholewheat pasta, brown rice and green peas, lentils and pulses.

UNDERSTANDING SUGAR

Sugar is a type of carbohydrate – you may hear sugar referred to as a 'simple' or 'fast-acting' carbohydrate. There are two main types of sugar:

➲ Naturally occurring sugars, such as those found in milk or fruit.

➲ Added sugar (also known as free sugars), such as those added to tinned fruit in heavy syrup, or used to make cakes, jams, biscuits, buns or fizzy drinks.

It is mainly these added sugars that we need to cut down on. They add energy in the form of calories to our diets but nothing else. Naturally occurring sugars, such as those found in fruit, usually come with some additional nutritional benefits, like vitamins and minerals. However, you need to be careful with fruit juices. They contain none or very little of the fibre that is found in a piece of fruit. Several pieces of fruit are needed to make one glass, so the energy in one glass is higher than in a single portion of fruit. Some have added sugars as well, so read the label. It's recommended that we stick to no more than one 150ml serving of fruit juice a day.

There are many different names for sugar – for example, table sugar, brown sugar, molasses, honey, beet sugar, cane sugar, icing sugar, raw sugar, maple syrup, high-fructose corn syrup, agave nectar and sugar cane syrup. You may also see table sugar listed by its chemical name, sucrose. Fruit sugar is also known as fructose and the sugar in milk is called lactose. If it ends with '–ose', then it is a sugar.

HOW MUCH SUGAR CAN WE EAT?

The government recommends that added sugars should not make up more than 5% of the calories you get from food and drink each day. This means:

➲ Adults should have no more than 30g added sugar a day (roughly equivalent to 7 sugar cubes).

➲ Children aged 7 to 10 should have no more than 24g added sugar a day (6 sugar cubes).

➲ Children aged 4 to 6 should have no more than 19g added sugar a day (5 sugar cubes).

➲ There is no guideline for children under the age of 4, but it is recommended that they avoid sugar-sweetened drinks and food with added sugar.

It is worth noting that choosing brown sugar instead of white makes no difference to the calorie content.

ARTIFICIAL SWEETENERS

Like sugar, sweeteners provide a sweet taste. What sets them apart is that, after consumption, they don't increase blood sugar levels. They are many times sweeter than sugar and can be an attractive alternative because they add virtually no calories to your diet. Also, you need only a fraction of the artificial sweetener, compared with the amount of sugar you would normally use, which is fortunate because they are generally a lot more expensive than sugar.

Stevia is one of the commonly used 'natural' ingredients in these products, and aspartame is another well-known chemical sweetener, but there are dozens of synthetic sugars used in a huge range of everyday products.

If you are struggling to do without fizzy drinks, you could switch to zero-calorie drinks, which contain artificial sweeteners instead of sugar, to help you kick the habit. These products may help to satisfy your craving without piling on the pounds. BUT, as with all things, it is best to use these artificial sweeteners in moderation, and the best advice is to cut back on sweet food and drinks generally. Water is by far the best thing to drink when you are trying to lose weight because it has no sugars in it and no calories. You should drink enough to quench your thirst and keep your urine a light colour, whether you are trying to lose weight or not.

Some of the recipes in this book use sugar or sweeteners, like honey, to improve taste. You could substitute these for an artificial sweetener in order to reduce your sugar and calorie intake, if required, though the end result might be a bit different.

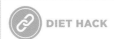 **DIET HACK**

Will fizzy diet drinks make me crave more sugar?
It has been suggested that the artificial sweeteners in diet fizzy drinks trigger the brain's sweetness receptors; the body then prepares itself for the influx of calories that come from sugar, but when that sugar doesn't come, the body still craves it and you may end up eating sugar-rich foods to deal with the craving. In fact, new research has revealed that, overall, dieters who drink zero-calorie fizzy drinks consume fewer calories and experience greater levels of weight loss. Ideally, however, we would use these drinks to wean ourselves off their full-sugar, full-fat cousins, and eventually switch to lightly flavoured or sparkling water – which will save you a fortune, too, since 1 litre of sparkling water costs a lot less than 1 litre of fizzy drinks!

UNDERSTANDING FIBRE

Fibre comes from plant foods including fruits, vegetables, whole grains, nuts and pulses. When you consume dietary fibre most of it passes through the intestines and is not digested. It contributes to digestive health, supports healthy gut bacteria, regulates blood sugar, helps to keep you regular and can make you feel full and satisfied after eating; it can also lower your cholesterol levels. For good health, adults need to try to eat 30g fibre each day, but many of us don't even come close. Make any changes to your diet gradually, especially when it comes to fibre, or you could experience discomfort or worse, embarrassment!

DIETARY FIBRE

Good sources of dietary fibre include:

➡ Peas, beans and pulses – such as black beans, kidney beans, pinto beans, chickpeas, white beans and lentils.

➡ Fruits and vegetables – especially those with edible skin, such as apples, corn and beans, and those with edible seeds, such as berries.

➡ Whole grains – such as wholewheat pasta, wholegrain breads and wholegrain cereals (check the label – you want 3g dietary fibre or more per serving), including those made from wholewheat, wheat bran and oats.

➡ Unsalted nuts and seeds – try different kinds. Peanuts, walnuts and almonds are a good source of fibre and healthy fat. But watch portion sizes because they are also high in calories, and check for added sugar.

➡ High-fibre products – e.g. certain yoghurts.

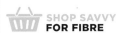
SHOP SAVVY
FOR FIBRE

Choose a high-fibre breakfast, such as porridge oats, which are also very cheap to buy. Swap your white loaf for wholemeal and add cheap pulses, like lentils, chickpeas and beans, to stews, curries and salads. Plenty of fibre in your diet can reduce the risk of heart disease, stroke and type 2 diabetes.

UNDERSTANDING SALT

Eating too much salt can raise your blood pressure, and having high-blood pressure puts added force against the walls of your arteries and makes your heart work harder. Over time this extra pressure can damage the arteries, which makes them more likely to become narrowed and hardened by fatty deposits. When this happens to your coronary arteries (the arteries that supply your heart muscle with oxygen-rich blood) it is called coronary heart disease, which can lead to angina and heart attack. Anyone can develop high blood pressure and it's very hard to tell if you have it because it rarely makes people feel ill. As a result, even if you think your blood pressure is fine, you should still limit the amount of salt you eat.

It is recommended that adults should eat no more than 6g salt a day – that's about one level teaspoon.

There is salt found in most processed foods so you need to pay attention to more than just the salt that you add to your meal during cooking or at the table. Around three quarters of the salt we eat has already been added to our food *before* we buy it. Things like bread, ready meals, packet sauces and breakfast cereals can all have high salt content. It's worth knowing that expensive sea salt and standard table salt are the same in terms of their effect on your body. Some food labels have a traffic light labelling system to help you to understand how much salt they contain:

HOW MUCH IS TOO MUCH PER 100G?

RED
high in salt
more than 1.5g
(more than
0.6g sodium)

AMBER
medium in salt
0.3–1.5g
(0.4–0.6g sodium)

GREEN
low in salt
0–0.3g
(0–0.1g sodium)

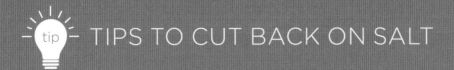

TIPS TO CUT BACK ON SALT

1 Try cooking without salt or adding less salt to your cooking when boiling vegetables and making casseroles and sauces.

2 Use spices and herbs to flavour foods rather than salt. This works really well, even with foods such as potatoes, pasta, rice and couscous.

3 Citrus fruits such as lemons and limes can add a zesty kick to fish, chicken and pork. Use them as a marinade with olive oil and garlic or simply squeeze the juices over your meal.

4 Watch out for cooking sauces (especially soy sauce) and ready-mixed 'seasonings' which can be very high in salt. If you're not sure how salty they are, check the label.

5 Choose low-salt stock cubes instead of the standard kind. They are not expensive and are a good resource if you are short on time. Watch out for cubes with a high potassium content – these are not good for people with type 2 diabetes/kidney disease.

6 Be careful with saltier foods, such as bacon and cheese. Avoid takeaways, ready meals and other processed foods.

7 If you do have to add salt, consider a low-sodium alternative. However, these may not be suitable for people with certain medical conditions (e.g. diabetes or kidney disease).

READING THE LABEL

Now you know how many calories you need to eat each day to achieve your safe and steady weight-loss goals (1,900 kcals/1,400 kcals per day for most men/women), you need to put all of this powerful knowledge about food groups to good use when you hit the supermarket. Some products will provide a calorie count for you on the label, which will help to keep you on track, but there are some other handy hints to help you shop smarter, too.

DAILY RECOMMENDED INTAKES FOR AN ADULT TO MAINTAIN A STABLE WEIGHT
(in other words, when you are not trying to lose weight)

- Energy:
  male 2,500 kcals
  female 2,000 kcals

- Total fat: less than 70g

- Saturates: less than 20g

- Carbohydrate: at least 260g

- Total sugars: 90g

- Protein: 50g

- Salt: less than 6g

(values for weight loss will be slightly less)

DOES IT REALLY DO EXACTLY WHAT IT SAYS ON THE TIN?

The nutritional labels on food and drinks look like the list below – but bear in mind that they are usually measured per 100g or per 100ml, which may be far less than the total size of the product. If the packet is actually 500g, for example, you will need to multiply the calories by five.

- **Energy (in kJ and kcals)** The amount of energy the food will give you when you eat it – this is the calorie count.

- **Fat (in g)** The total amount of fat contained in the food. On a normal diet of 2,000 kcals for a woman and 2,500 kcals for a man, no more than 70g/95g of your food per day should come from fats.

- **Saturates (in g)** You want to eat less of these and look for unsaturated fats instead.

- **Carbohydrates (in g)** Go for complex fibre-rich carbs when you can.

- **Sugars (in g)** Choose lower sugar options whenever possible.

- **Protein (in g)** You should aim for 50g per day.

- **Salt (in g)** Eat no more than 6g per day – that's just a teaspoon.

How can you tell by looking at the label if a food is really high in fat, saturated fat, sugars or salt?

FAT

HIGH IN FAT –
MORE THAN 17.5G FAT
PER 100G

LOW IN FAT –
3G FAT OR LESS
PER 100G

**SATURATED FAT
(SATURATES)**

HIGH IN SATURATES –
MORE THAN 5G SATURATES
PER 100G

LOW IN SATURATES –
1.5G SATURATES OR
LESS PER 100G

SUGARS

HIGH IN SUGARS –
MORE THAN 22.5G TOTAL
SUGARS PER 100G

LOW IN SUGARS –
5G TOTAL SUGARS
OR LESS PER 100G

SALT

HIGH IN SALT –
MORE THAN 1.5G SALT
PER 100G

LOW IN SALT –
0.3G SALT OR
LESS PER 100G

LOW-FAT AND 'LITE' PRODUCTS

Obviously, when it comes to saving money and losing weight, you want to avoid wasting your cash on products that don't live up to the hype. This is especially true when it comes to products that claim to be low in sugar, fats or calories. We regularly test these products in the series and often find that there are negligible benefits in paying more money for these foods. By taking control and reading the labels you will discover that it is portion size that often makes the difference.

To say that a food is 'light' or 'lite', it must be at least 30% lower in calories or fat than standard products. The easiest way to compare them is to look at the amount of fat or kcals per 100g. It may surprise you to know that a 'light' or 'lite' version of one brand of crisps may contain the same amount of fat or calories per 100g as the standard version – some actually just put fewer crisps in a smaller bag! In this case, you would be better off buying the normal, cheaper crisps and eating half a bag. (Admittedly, that is going to be the tricky part!) Also, be wary of some low-fat products as the fat may have been replaced with sugar.

Remember, the manufacturer's idea of what constitutes a 'serving' or a 'portion' might not be the same as yours. Stick to your own calorie count, or use the calorie info per 100g, and work it out for yourself.

To reduce the calorie content in foods, such as low-fat ice cream, the manufacturers usually have to replace the fats with lots of sweeteners, which can cause digestive discomfort. It might be better in health cost and calorie terms to have just a little bit less of the normal brands.

Watch out for foods that claim to have added protein or claim to be low carb. Read the labels and you will often discover that your usual brand of bread, for instance, hasn't got much more carbohydrate than the low-carb version. You may also be able to switch to a cheaper wholegrain loaf, which would do the same job. Sausage brands often offer low-salt or higher protein options but swapping to turkey or chicken sausages would be healthier and cheaper.

SAVVY SHOPPING TIPS

1 Always use a shopping list – it will help you to separate your needs from your wants.

2 Don't shop when you are hungry or on an empty stomach; you'll end up buying things you don't need.

3 An online delivery can cost as little as £1 and if it stops you making unhealthy impulse buys in store then it may be worth it – and you can keep an eye on your total spend as you go.

4 Take advantage of deals and BOGOFs to stock your freezer. And bear in mind that frozen veggies and fish are often much cheaper than their fresh cousins.

5 Always try own brands and use low-cost supermarkets to bag nutritious bargains.

6 Batch-cooked food and healthy, low-calorie meals will be easy to grab and go.

7 Go low – many of the healthiest and cheapest foods in your supermarket are not at eye level. Look down to lower shelves to bag the bargains.

8 Check out the reduced-price section in your supermarket. You can pick up some great bargains there – just freeze anything that you can't use on the day you buy it.

9 Save money on your favourite produce by looking in the freezer aisle all year round. Frozen fruits and veggies, which are picked and prepped at their prime, can be even more nutritious than the fresh stuff. Just steer clear of anything with added sugar, syrups or sauces.

10 Do most of your shopping in the outside aisles – this is where you'll find the fresh foods in the majority of main-stream supermarkets. Once you start venturing into the middle aisles, the nutrients go down and the calorie load goes up!

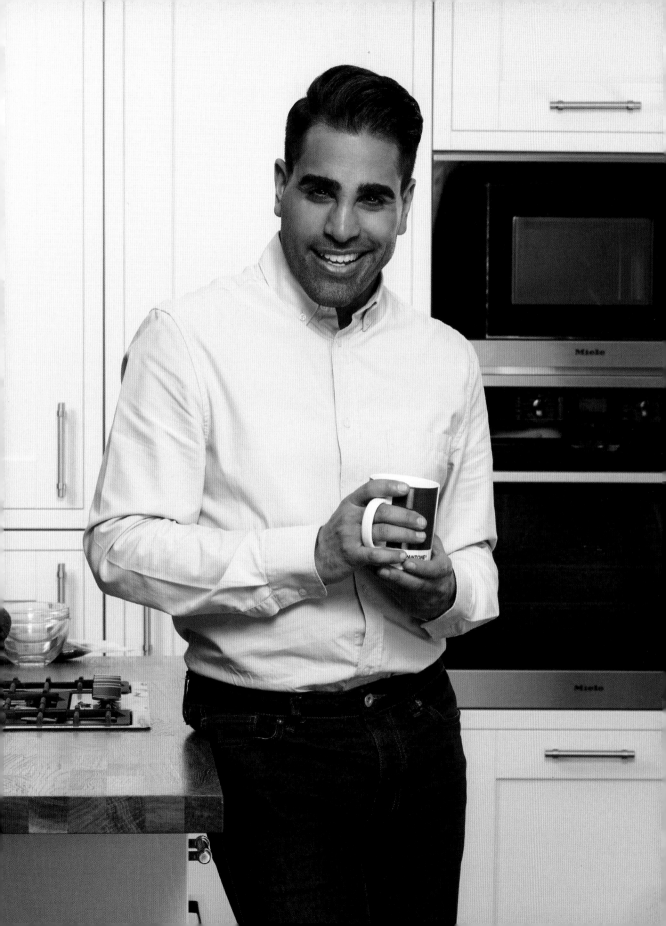

LOW-COST EXERCISE

I'm not tall, so when I put on weight, my BMI goes into the overweight category very quickly. I know that exercise will help and so I try my best to get out and do it. A big motivator for me is meeting up with friends to exercise, because then I know that I have to show up. It's very hard to shirk if someone is depending on you!

GETTING STARTED

First of all, if you currently don't do any exercise, think about why you aren't managing to get down to it. If necessary, ask yourself the motivational questions again (see page 19). If you haven't exercised for a long time or are out of shape, you can start by making sure

CALORIE-BURNING CHART FOR VARIOUS ACTIVITIES
Approximate kcals burned, per hour, by a 68kg (10 stone 7lb) woman

Exercise	kcals/hour	Exercise	kcals/hour
Sleeping	55	Skating/blading	420+
Eating	85	Dancing, aerobic	420+
Sewing/knitting	85	Aerobics	450+
Sitting	85	Bicycling, moderate	450+
Standing	100	Jogging, 5mph	500+
Driving	110	Gardening, digging	500+
Office work	140	Swimming, active	500+
Golf, with a trolley	180	Cross-country ski machine	500+
Golf, without a trolley	240	Hiking	500+
Gardening, planting	250	Step aerobics	550+
Dancing, ballroom	260	Rowing	550+
Walking, 3mph	280+	Power walking	600+
Table tennis	290+	Cycling, studio	650
Gardening, hoeing etc.	350+	Squash	650+
Tennis	350+	Skipping with rope	700+
Water aerobics	400+	Running	700+

you walk for at least 30 minutes each day and gradually build up from there. If you try this alongside the calorie-controlled meal plans (see pages 210–16), I'm sure you'll notice a difference by the end of the four weeks. If you are really struggling, start small and increase your time each week, e.g. walk for 10 minutes a day in week one, then 20 minutes a day in week two and so on.

IT'S A SIMPLE EQUATION:

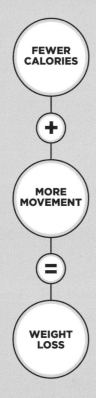

FEWER CALORIES

+

MORE MOVEMENT

=

WEIGHT LOSS

The good news is that many of our dieters on the series experienced a huge surge of energy just a week or two into their healthy-eating plans, as their body adjusted to the fabulous new fuel it was getting. You will feel more like exercising as soon as your healthy-eating plans kick in – and exercise also reduces the hormones linked to stress. It's a win, win.

There are many low- and no-cost ways to burn calories and, in order to improve your weight-loss chances, you really need to get moving. It's not always about planned exercise either; it can be just as much about incorporating activity into your daily routine. Move more and your body will burn more calories. One of our dieters from the series who had always taken the lift at work in the past, became 'the stair master' and noticed great results, even claiming she had 'lost a chin' in the process!

Exercise is predominately for fitness and is a great way to boost your metabolism. When our bodies have more muscle, we metabolise food and burn calories far more efficiently. Expensive gym memberships are not necessary to achieve these things, though, as there are lots of low- or no-cost options available. Your local council will have information on the free activities that are happening near you. It's also worth checking with your GP.

There is a big move towards 'social prescribing' at the moment because studies show that 20% of patients consult their GP with problems that could be solved by better connections to community services and social interaction, and your local surgery will have details of any dance and exercise groups that are meeting up near you.

Understandably, some of us feel self-conscious, especially if we haven't exercised in a while, and you may prefer to exercise at home to begin with. There are still lots of ways that you can squeeze those vital minutes of exercise into your normal routine, though. There are lots of free exercise videos online for a start! Remember, stronger bodies with more muscle metabolise food better.

REALISTIC EXERCISE GOALS

The current UK government recommendation for 19–64-year-olds is at least 150 minutes of moderate aerobic activity a week (e.g. cycling/brisk walking), as well as strength exercises on 2 or more days a week (e.g. weights, resistance bands, gardening or yoga). Just walking at a normal pace for 30 minutes will burn a minimum of 140 kcals for most people, and you will feel great afterwards. And you don't need to buy expensive kit – you could use some tins of beans as weights and an old pair of stretchy leggings or tights to create your own resistance bands instead. Simply hold the fabric in each hand and stretch it as you extend your arms apart, giving your arms and chest a workout.

In just 28 days you will be amazed how much you can achieve for little or no cost.

START SMALL – AT HOME

Exercising in the privacy of your own home can be a brilliant way to build confidence. Many of the most popular exercise DVDs are available cheaply from your local charity shop if you need a bit of encouragement and variety.

The more you exercise, the more energy you will have. As your fitness grows why not add a brisk walk to the shops into your routine? Playing with your children, cleaning and gardening are also brilliant ways to burn extra calories and, as you get stronger and fitter, you will want to do these things on top of your daily half hour of exercise.

INCIDENTAL EXERCISE AROUND THE HOUSE

As well as deliberate exercise, which is really important, I love 'incidental' exercise. I have a friend who always does squats when she brushes her teeth. It's part of her routine now and because she would never skip brushing her teeth, the squats always get done, too. Smaller bursts of exercise like this can work well. When you are feeling fit enough, you could try doing the plank three times a day when you are at home; although, I have heard of teams of co-workers doing the plank together in the office as well. Keep light hand weights or a bottle of water handy while you watch TV. Just raise it up and down during your favourite programme and you will be giving your biceps a workout.

If you wouldn't know where to begin with the plank and you don't know your squats from a squash, then the internet offers an endless supply of free exercise videos with useful demonstrations to help you mix up your exercise plans.

BRANCH OUT – INTO THE GREAT OUTDOORS

Like many people, I have to be indoors for work, so I think exercising in the outdoors is great if you can manage it. Wind resistance and negotiating uneven ground and hills makes your body work harder, too. The environment is constantly changing so you won't get bored and parks are packed with equipment that you can use. So much of the exercise we can do outdoors is free. Parkruns, a collection of 5km runs that take place all over the country, cater for all levels of fitness and are a great way to meet like-minded people. The Daily Mile initiative for kids gets them outside walking or jogging for 15 minutes every day. You can find lots of free 'Couch to 5K' plans that get you walking and enjoying the benefits of aerobic exercise. You could build up to running but, even if you don't, the important thing is that you are still exercising, burning more calories and getting outside is good for your mental health.

TECHNOLOGY AND THE INTERNET

There are lots of free apps that you can download to track how much you move in a day. Step counters start at just a couple of pounds and they can really help to remind you to move more. Some of our phones have the capacity to track exercise and that costs nothing – use the tools you have already.

SHAKE A TAIL FEATHER

To commit to exercise it will help if you find something that you love doing. I found out relatively recently that I love dancing. I was really surprised, which shows that we should take a chance on new things – you might just discover something that could change your attitude to exercise for life.

Dancing helped me to lose weight but it also increases muscle strength, endurance and aerobic fitness, and it improves coordination, agility and flexibility. You can keep dancing for years, well into old age, and it might help to improve your memory as well.

Lessons can cost as little as £5 and, when you're up and running, you can go to the many free social dancing sessions that happen at weekends and in the evenings.

If dancing isn't your thing, walking will work just as well. Make a playlist! Choose your favourite music, or download some free podcasts and audiobooks, and you can expand your mind as you shrink your waistline.

INCIDENTAL EXERCISE AT WORK

Some of the simplest forms of incidental exercise can be incorporated into your normal day at work. Lots of people suggest taking the stairs but even that can seem quite ambitious and very public if you are just starting out. And, let's face it, who wants to be sweaty and exhausted at work? Start gently – take the stairs down and use the lift to go up until you can manage both.

Alternating between sitting and standing at work is also really important. Every 20–30 minutes change your position because this will use up calories. Many work places now offer desks that enable you to stand up all day, too. It's also a great idea to get away from your desk at lunch time. If possible, go for a walk every day – the psychological and physical benefits are huge.

Why must we always have meetings sitting down with biscuits? The next time you arrange to meet, have a walking meeting instead. And try stand-up meetings at work – your colleagues might thank you and you could find it keeps the meetings shorter, as well!

RECIPES

Diets can feel isolating if you are eating low-calorie meals for one. Your chances of success will improve greatly if you can eat the same food as your family. These recipes have been devised with this in mind and all are economical, quick to make and require no fancy equipment. Preparing and cooking this fabulous food together means that no one will be left out. Why not make the nutritious smoothies for breakfast? Or try the family-friendly midweek suppers, like Five Vegetable Lasagne on page 129 or Turkey Meatballs with Tomato Sauce on page 136? You will be making healthier food choices for everyone. There are recipes particularly suited to batch cooking, too, which makes it even easier to have family-friendly, low-cost and delicious foods ready in no time. Try Lentil & Tomato Bolognaise on page 134 or Sausage Ragu with Brown Rice on page 160 – double up the quantities and freeze leftover portions for another week.

Socialising around food is also important, so why not rustle up the Mexican-style Eggs on page 68 for a grown-up weekend brunch? In my opinion, if you have been keeping to your optimal calorie intake all week, then you should be able to have a dessert at the weekend. The recipe for the (not-too-naughty) Gooey Dark Chocolate Pots on page 179 ticks all of the boxes for me! These low-calorie spins on classic favourites will make your diet feel flexible and more manageable and, dare I say it, more fun – we've even included a low-calorie tipple or two.

I have battled to change my eating habits for years. As a paediatrician I know that your early food habits can set a pattern for life. It was that way for me. Although certain diets (see pages 12–14) can work in the short term, as a doctor, I advocate a balanced, calorie-controlled and varied diet as the best way of maintaining long-term good health and weight. There's no better way of achieving this than cooking simple, interesting and varied dishes. Some of the breakfast recipes serve two, since the family might not all want to eat the same thing every day, but most mains serve four. A couple of the puddings serve six – you can freeze these so you're not tempted to indulge.

While all of these recipes are perfect to share with your family, very young children, older relatives and those with certain medical conditions will have extra dietary needs that you should consider, too.

CHILDREN AND NUTRITION

The health of children is a subject that is very close to my heart. Children are not just 'mini adults' and certain nutrients, like protein, iron and calcium, are especially important at certain times to support their growth and development. At the same time, it is clear from the figures available that young children's diets are providing more sugary energy than they actually need, and they still aren't getting the fruit, vegetables, oily fish and fibre that they should be.

Levels of childhood obesity in England are among the highest in the developed world, with almost 1 in 4 children being overweight or obese before starting school. Children who are overweight or obese in childhood are more likely to become obese adults; this often leads to long-term health issues, including heart disease, type 2 diabetes and some cancers. Unless a child is significantly overweight, though, I would not recommend a 'diet' – healthier eating and physical activity should be the norm!

THE LATEST NATIONAL DIET AND NUTRITION SURVEY (NDNS) FIGURES

↻ Sugar makes up 13.5% of the daily calorie intake of 4- to 10-year-olds and 14.1% of teenagers (11- to 18-year-olds) ; the official recommendation is to limit sugar to no more than 5%.

↻ Sugary drink intake is more than double in teenagers than in younger children (191g), even though consumption has decreased by 30%; sugary drinks remain the main source of sugar (22%) in their diets.

OLDER PEOPLE

Older people need to try and eat a healthy, balanced diet, and for some individuals a calorie-restricted or low-fat diet can be extremely harmful. Being underweight is as dangerous as being overweight for older people. In fact, as we age we need to choose food rich in vitamins and minerals, as low levels of vitamin D, B12, iron and vitamin C have been found in surveys of older people. Individuals with unplanned weight loss will also need to consume food that is higher in fat and protein, like full-fat milk, cheese and cream, which flies in the face of all of the healthy-eating guidance.

It is a myth that losing weight and becoming frail is an inevitable part of ageing but around 1 in 10 older people in the UK are malnourished or at risk of malnutrition – that's around 1 million older people. Malnutrition is a major cause and consequence of poor health, and older people are particularly vulnerable. Loss of appetite is common in older adults and, as we age, the body doesn't feel the signals for hunger or thirst as much. This means that some older people don't recognise their needs. Good nutrition helps us to age well and stay fitter and healthier for longer. Nutrition also plays a large role in cognitive function, protecting us from life-limiting conditions. While the majority of healthy-eating advice is right for the general population or younger audiences, it may not be suitable for older populations.

KEY TO SYMBOLS

 Batch cook & freeze

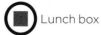 Lunch box

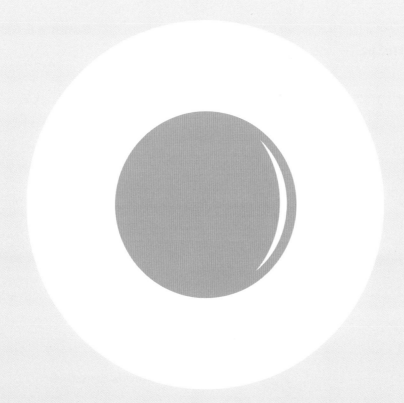

BREAKFAST

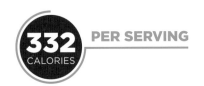
332 CALORIES | PER SERVING

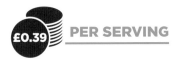
£0.39 | PER SERVING

CHOCOLATE ORANGE PORRIDGE
SERVES 2

This is a really easy but delicious way to jazz up your ordinary porridge, a real chocolatey hit with little ones too. A cheap but nutritious way to fill you up before a busy day. (Also pictured is **Banana & Cinnamon Porridge**, recipe on page 56.)

100g porridge oats
200ml semi-skimmed milk
1 orange
1 tbsp cocoa powder
2 tsp honey

1 In a saucepan, bring the oats, milk and 300ml water to a light simmer over a medium heat.

2 Zest the orange and stir the zest into the porridge. Reduce the heat and simmer gently for 10 minutes.

3 Meanwhile, cut the skin off the orange and cut into bite-sized pieces.

4 Just before serving, stir the cocoa powder through the porridge.

5 Spoon into bowls and top with the orange pieces and drizzle with a little bit of honey to serve.

DIET HACK
Can you eat chocolate for breakfast?

A recent study found that a group of people who ate a 600-kcal breakfast each day, including a slice of chocolate cake, lost more weight than those who had a 300-kcal low-carb breakfast. Now, I'm not recommending you eat chocolate cake but you do need to think of your body like a car. Fuel yourself when you plan to be moving and not when you're parked. The breakfast in this study also included protein, so why not try the Quick Banana & Oat Pancakes (see page 62) with a teaspoon of chocolate spread – you'll have had a balanced breakfast with a sweat treat in the mix. Remember – people who skip breakfast are 30% more likely to be obese.

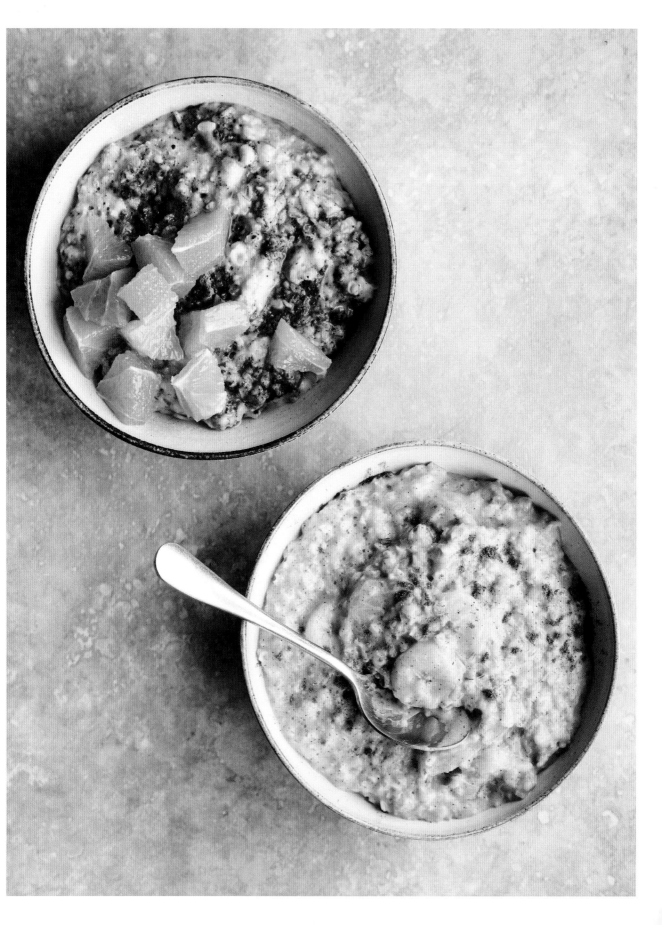

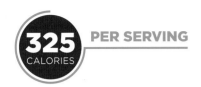 **PER SERVING**

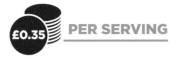 **PER SERVING**

BANANA & CINNAMON PORRIDGE
SERVES 2

Porridge is undoubtedly a great way to start your day – inexpensive, packed full of fibre, quick and filling. The banana and cinnamon here add a great warmth and sweetness. (See photo on previous page.)

100g porridge oats
200ml semi-skimmed milk
1 banana, sliced
1 tsp ground cinnamon

1 In a saucepan, bring the oats, milk and 300ml water to a light simmer over a medium heat.

2 Add the sliced banana and cinnamon, reduce the heat and simmer gently for 10 minutes, stirring regularly.

3 Spoon into bowls to serve.

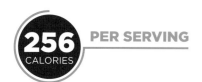
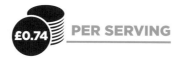

SPICED APPLE OVERNIGHT OATS
SERVES 2

This is a great midweek breakfast option – you prepare it all the night before and it is ready and waiting for you in the morning. Perfect for taking into work.

50g porridge oats
2 apples, cored and grated
1 tsp ground cinnamon
1 tbsp honey
1 tsp vanilla extract
100g natural yoghurt
Splash of semi-skimmed
 milk, to serve

1 Combine all of the ingredients, except the milk, together in a bowl and mix well. Cover and leave in the fridge overnight.

2 Just before serving, stir in a splash of milk to loosen the oats to your desired consistency.

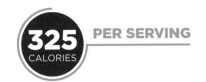
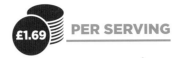
OAT, BERRY & COCONUT SMOOTHIE
SERVES 2

Smoothies are a brilliant midweek breakfast option, particularly good for on the go. You can cram in lots of goodness and often get children to eat fruit and vegetables that they wouldn't otherwise touch. Frozen berries are a great ingredient to have in your freezer, much cheaper than fresh berries and infinitely more tasty when the fresh ones aren't in season. Frozen berries are also great stirred through porridge. This can make a good snack if you have a sweet craving but don't want to blow your calorie intake. (Also pictured are **Green Smoothie**, recipe on page 60, and **Tropical Citrus Smoothie**, recipe on page 61.)

175g frozen berries
100g natural yoghurt
1 × 400ml tin coconut milk
25g porridge oats

1 Whizz all the ingredients together in a blender until smooth.

2 Pour into glasses to serve.

AVOID SKIPPING MEALS
Try not to skip breakfast as this can make you feel tired and hungry and more likely to reach for high-fat, high-sugar snacks later on. A good brekkie will improve your concentration throughout the morning, too.

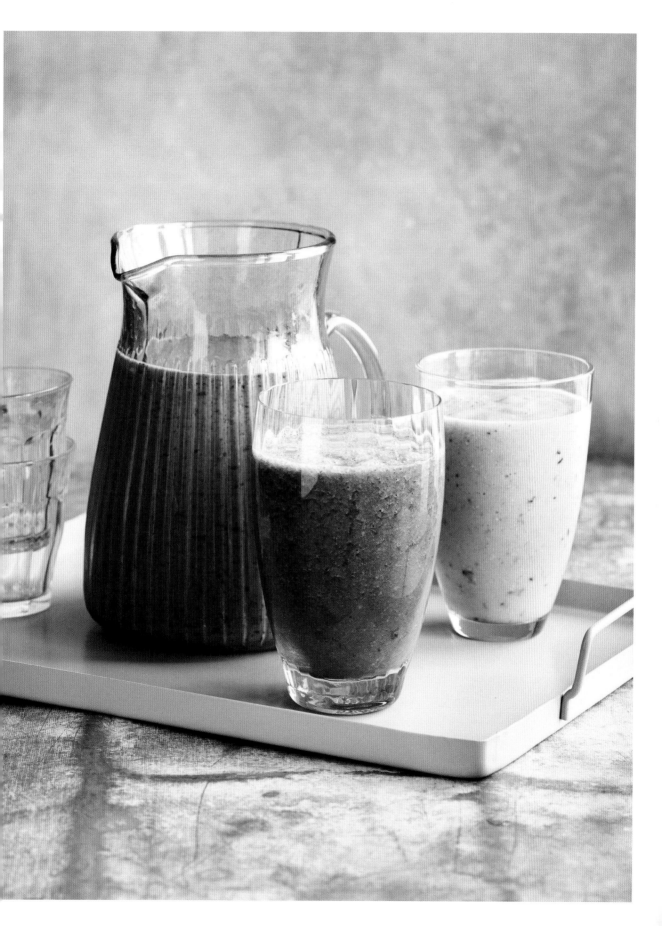

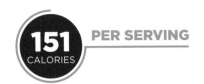 **151 CALORIES** | **PER SERVING**

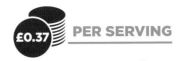 **£0.37** | **PER SERVING**

GREEN SMOOTHIE
SERVES 2

This is a great smoothie recipe and a really good way of getting some leafy greens into your diet. Frozen spinach is a wonder ingredient – inexpensive, readily available and it's so handy to have a stash in the freezer for times when you are out of fresh vegetables. You can use fresh spinach if you have some – just add a few ice cubes to the blender if you do. (See photo on previous page.)

100g frozen spinach
1 banana
½ avocado

1 Place all the ingredients in a blender with 300ml water and whizz until smooth.

2 Pour into glasses to serve.

MAKE DIY SMOOTHIE AND SALAD PACKS
I'm not a fan of food prep, so when I chop up fruit for smoothies, I make enough for a few days and divide it up into smoothie portions. I'll store them in sandwich bags or food storage boxes and put them in the freezer. It cuts down on waste and saves money and hassle. The same works for salad bags – except you should store those in the fridge. (You can reuse the sandwich bags – just wash them out, then leave to dry.)

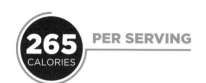
265 CALORIES PER SERVING

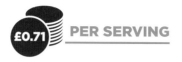
£0.71 PER SERVING

TROPICAL CITRUS SMOOTHIE
SERVES 2

Most big supermarkets sell bags of frozen tropical fruit that include things like mangoes, papaya, pineapple and melons. Frozen fruit is a great alternative to fresh – it's cheaper and means less waste as you just use what you need, rather than having half a melon lingering at the back of the fridge. (See photo on page 59.)

2 oranges, peeled
175g frozen tropical fruit
200ml almond milk
   (or other dairy/non-dairy
   milk or water)
25g porridge oats
1 banana

1 Whizz all the ingredients together in a blender until smooth.

2 Pour into glasses to serve.

309 CALORIES **PER SERVING**

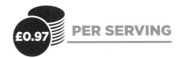

£0.97 **PER SERVING**

QUICK BANANA & OAT PANCAKES

SERVES 4

Being able to eat pancakes for breakfast when you are trying to lose weight is a real joy! These are quick and easy to make and will be a hit with the whole family. Try different toppings according to your calorie allowance – extra fruit or a compote made from frozen fruit would both be particularly delicious spooned over the top.

4 bananas, mashed
4 eggs
100g porridge oats
Pinch of ground cinnamon
2 tsp vegetable oil or
   unsalted butter
4 tbsp natural yoghurt,
   to serve

1 In a small bowl, combine the mashed bananas, eggs, oats and cinnamon and mix well.

2 Heat half the oil or butter in a frying pan over a medium heat. Spoon tablespoonfuls of the mixture into the pan and fry the pancakes for 2–4 minutes on each side, or until golden brown and cooked through. Repeat with the remaining mixture, adding more oil or butter to the pan if necessary, to make 4–6 pancakes per person.

3 Serve with the yoghurt.

🛒 **SHOP SAVVY** LOW-FAT PLAIN YOGHURT

A cut-price source of protein and a great alternative to sugary breakfast cereal, yoghurt can also contain bacteria that benefit the digestive tract. Try mixing it with some low-cost, frozen blueberries for a high-protein snack, or use it instead of sour cream in just about any recipe – it will help lower the calorie content of your dish and boost the protein. Stick to a plain yoghurt with the fewest ingredients and sugars, and avoid added flavours because these always mean more added sugar. If you want to add your own honey, restrict yourself to a teaspoon.

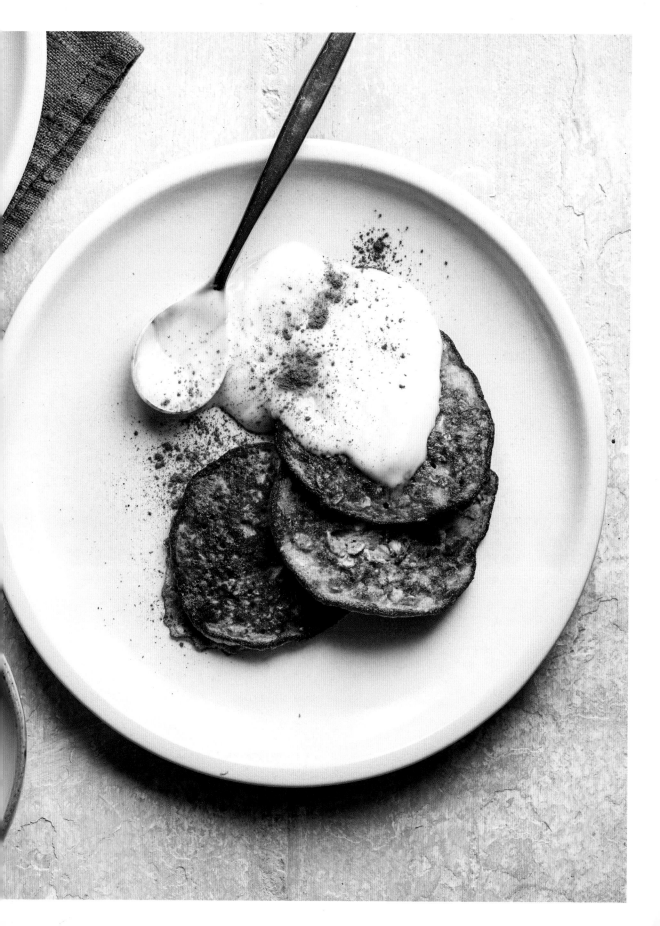

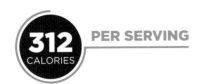 **PER SERVING**

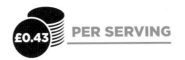 **PER SERVING**

SPINACH & EGG FRENCH TOAST
SERVES 4

This is a great weekend breakfast for the whole family and feels like a nice treat, too. It's a really simple recipe and is an ideal one for getting some extra greens in your diet. It's a delicious Sunday night dinner when you can't face cooking a full meal. This is best made with a good, brown seeded bread – make sure you soak the bread properly in the egg and spinach mixture.

170g frozen spinach
8 eggs
8 slices bread
2 tsp unsalted butter
2 tsp vegetable oil

 DIET HACK
Make Your Own Oil Spray
It can be hard to judge the amount of oil that you need to put in a pan and oils can be very calorific. Why not make your own spray? Add 4 parts distilled water (water that has been boiled and cooled) to 1 part oil of your choice to a clean spray bottle. Shake well and you have a free way of controlling how much oil you use.

1 Defrost the spinach – either in the microwave (place in a bowl and cook on high for 1–2 minutes) or place in a sieve over the sink and pour boiling water over the top. Squeeze and drain out the excess water.

2 Place the spinach in a bowl and crack in the eggs. Whisk everything together with a fork.

3 Soak the slices of bread in the spinach and egg mix one at a time, turning them over to ensure both sides are coated and well soaked.

4 Meanwhile, place a frying pan over a medium heat. Add half the butter and oil, then add a few slices of the soaked bread and fry for 3 minutes on each side, or until golden brown. Add the remaining butter and oil to the pan and repeat with the remaining slices.

5 Serve straight from the pan.

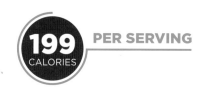

199 CALORIES PER SERVING

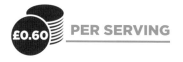

£0.60 PER SERVING

QUICK MUSHROOM & TOMATO BREAKFAST SCRAMBLE
SERVES 2

Adding chopped veg to your scrambled eggs is a great way to fill up on the good stuff first thing in the morning – and it will stop you reaching for a slice of toast. You can use any vegetables here – use up what you have in the fridge, rather than buying more. Chopped courgette, avocado, peppers or spinach would also be delicious.

4 eggs
2 tsp unsalted butter
100g cherry tomatoes, halved
100g mushrooms, sliced

1 Whisk the eggs in a small bowl and set aside.

2 Melt the butter in a non-stick saucepan over a medium to high heat. Add the tomatoes and mushrooms and cook for 5 minutes until the mushrooms are brown and the tomatoes are soft.

3 Stir in the egg and scramble just long enough for the eggs to cook. Serve immediately.

🧺 **SHOP SAVVY** EGGS

Eggs are one of the cheapest and most nutrient-dense foods. Just one large egg contains 6g protein. They are filling because this high-quality protein satisfies the appetite, providing all the essential amino acids. Several studies have shown that having eggs for breakfast helps keep hunger at bay, which means you crave fewer calories throughout the day.

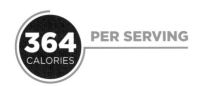

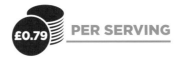

SWEETCORN FRITTERS WITH POACHED EGGS

SERVES 4

Sweetcorn is a good store cupboard staple and these fritters are a great go-to recipe when you don't have much in the fridge. These fritters are perfect for a weekend brunch but also good for lunch or a light dinner, too. They freeze really well – just stack them in between sheets of baking parchment for easy defrosting. They are very popular with kids (omit the coriander and spring onion if yours are averse to either).

2 × 198g tins low-salt sweetcorn, drained
100g self-raising flour
1 bunch of spring onions, finely sliced
15g fresh coriander, finely chopped
8 eggs
1 tbsp vegetable oil
Black pepper

1 Place the sweetcorn, flour, spring onions and coriander in a bowl, crack in four of the eggs and mix everything together until it forms a sticky batter.

2 Heat the oil in a frying pan and fry tablespoonfuls of the sweetcorn mixture for 2 minutes on each side, until golden brown and cooked through. Transfer to a plate and keep warm in a low oven, while you cook the remaining fritters.

3 Meanwhile, bring a large pan of water to a light simmer. Crack the remaining eggs into four separate mugs and gently tip them into the simmering water. Cook gently for 3–4 minutes before removing the eggs with a slotted spoon.

4 Divide the fritters between four plates, top each pile with a poached egg and sprinkle of black pepper and serve.

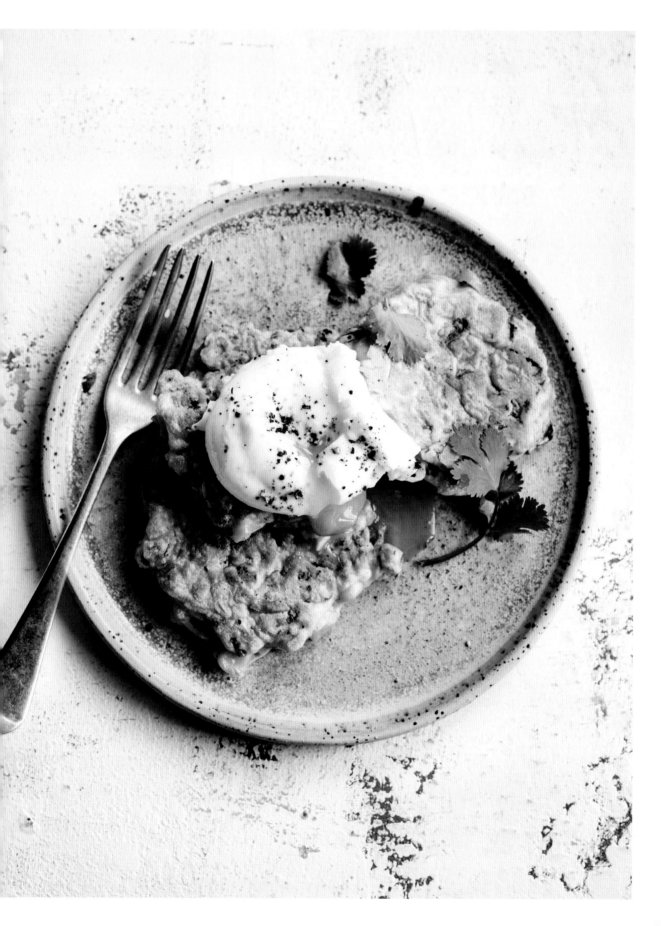

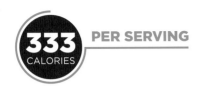 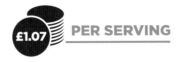

MEXICAN-STYLE EGGS
SERVES 4

This is a lovely weekend brunch recipe that is packed full of punchy Mexican flavours with loads of nutrient-rich ingredients. Ditch the chilli if you are cooking for kids and adjust the cooking time depending on whether you like eggs runny or more well done. Use any feta that is leftover in the packet as a filling for the Spinach Wraps (see page 88) or in a frittata.

1 tbsp olive oil
1 red onion, finely chopped
1 red pepper, sliced
3 cloves garlic,
    finely chopped
2 tsp smoked paprika
2 × 400g tins chopped
    tomatoes
Pinch of chilli flakes
    (optional)
4 eggs
1 avocado, sliced
75g feta, crumbled
30g fresh coriander,
    chopped
Black pepper

1 Heat the oil in a large casserole pan (one that has a lid) over a medium heat. Add the onion and pepper and sauté for 5 minutes. Stir in the garlic and paprika and cook for a further 2–3 minutes, stirring regularly to ensure it doesn't burn.

2 Add the tinned tomatoes, chilli flakes (if using) and season with black pepper. Reduce the heat and leave to simmer for 15 minutes.

3 Make 4 slight dips in the sauce using the back of a spoon and crack an egg into each dip – it's easier to crack the eggs into a mug or small bowl first then pour them in gently. Cover the pan with a lid and cook for 5–10 minutes until the whites are set but the yolks are still runny (cook for another 5 minutes if you prefer the yolks cooked through).

4 Remove the pan from the heat, place the avocado slices on top then scatter with the feta and coriander before serving.

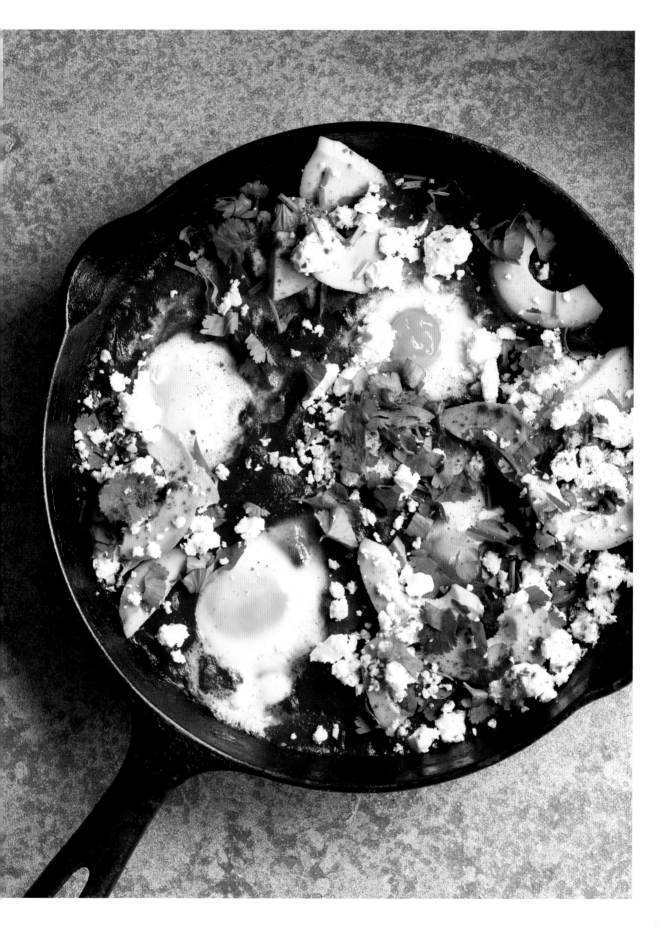

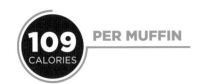
109 CALORIES — **PER MUFFIN**

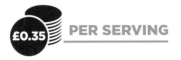
£0.35 **PER SERVING**

EGG, BACON & SPINACH BREAKFAST MUFFINS

MAKES 8–10 MUFFINS

Eggs are a really brilliant food for breakfast as they're packed with nutrients, quick to cook, cheap and versatile. These muffins are perfect for those mornings when you don't have much time – make up the batter the night before, store it in the fridge, then bake the muffins when you wake up. They're best eaten warm but they also freeze well.

4 rashers unsmoked
   streaky bacon,
   roughly chopped
4 eggs
50ml vegetable oil
15g fresh chives, snipped
85g frozen spinach
75g self-raising flour
½ tsp baking powder
Black pepper

1 Preheat the oven to 200°C/Fan 180°C and line a muffin tin with paper cases.

2 Fry the bacon over a medium heat in a non-stick pan for 10 minutes, or until starting to crisp up. Remove from the heat and set aside to cool.

3 Crack the eggs into a mixing bowl, add the oil and chives, season with black pepper and whisk together until combined.

4 Defrost the spinach – either in the microwave (place in a bowl and cook on high for 1–2 minutes) or place in a sieve over the sink and pour boiling water over the top. Drain and squeeze out any excess water.

5 Add the spinach and bacon to the bowl and mix well. Finally, sift the flour and baking powder into the bowl and fold in until fully combined.

6 Spoon the mixture into each case and bake in the oven for 15 minutes.

7 Leave to cool slightly on a wire rack. Best eaten as soon after baking as possible.

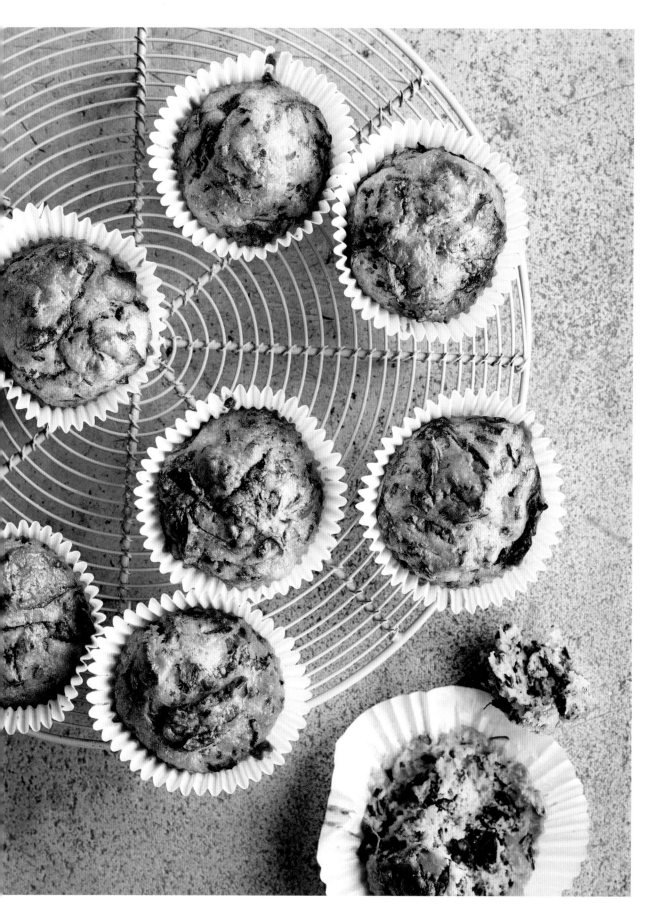

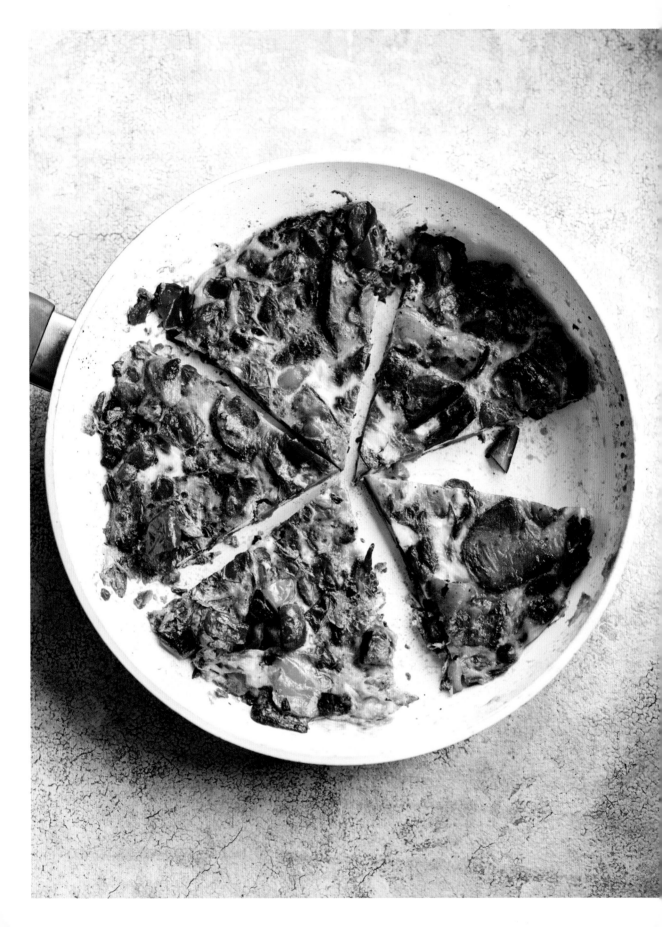

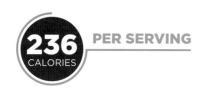
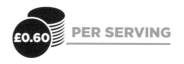
EASY FRIDGE RAID OMELETTE

SERVES 2

Omelettes are really versatile (and cheap to make) and this recipe is designed to use up those odds and ends of vegetables you might have lurking in your fridge. Use a good non-stick pan and add a little grated Cheddar or crumbled feta if you have the calorie allowance.

350g vegetables, finely chopped (use some or a mixture of carrots, onions, mushrooms, peppers, courgette and broccoli – whatever you have in your fridge!)
4 tsp vegetable oil
4 eggs
15g fresh soft herbs, finely chopped (use one or a mixture of parsley, coriander, dill and basil), or 1 tsp dried mixed herbs
Black pepper

1 Preheat the oven to 200°C/Fan 180°C.

2 Place the chopped vegetables in a roasting tin and drizzle with 2 teaspoons of the oil. Roast in the oven for 30–35 minutes.

3 Once the vegetables are roasted, whisk the eggs in a small bowl, add the chopped herbs and season with black pepper.

4 Heat the remaining oil in a frying pan over a medium heat. Pour in the egg mixture, swirling the eggs with a wooden spoon as they start to set. Tip your roasted veg on top of the eggs, spreading them out evenly. Leave to cook in the pan until just set.

5 Divide between two plates and serve.

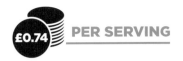
VEGETABLE FRITTERS WITH GARLIC ROAST TOMATOES
SERVES 4

This is a really quick and delicious way to get lots of vegetables into your diet. You can prepare these in advance and keep them warm in a low oven, or make a batch and freeze them between sheets of baking parchment. For extra protein, top with poached eggs or crumbled feta, though this will, of course, increase the calories.

600g cherry tomatoes, halved
2 tbsp vegetable oil
6 cloves garlic
2 courgettes, coarsely grated (approx. 300g)
2 carrots, coarsely grated (approx. 150g)
2 eggs, beaten
50g self-raising flour
Black pepper

1 Preheat the oven to 200°C/Fan 180°C.

2 Place the tomatoes in a roasting tin and drizzle with 1 tablespoon of the oil. Add the garlic (whole with the skins still on) and roast for 30 minutes. Remove from the oven, squeeze the cooked garlic from their skins and mix through the roast tomatoes.

3 Meanwhile, place the courgette and carrot in a bowl with the eggs and flour. Season with black pepper and mix until everything is combined.

4 Heat the remaining oil in a frying pan over a medium heat and cook spoonfuls of the mixture for 3–4 minutes on each side, until golden brown and cooked through.

5 Divide the fritters between four plates and top with the garlicky, roasted tomatoes.

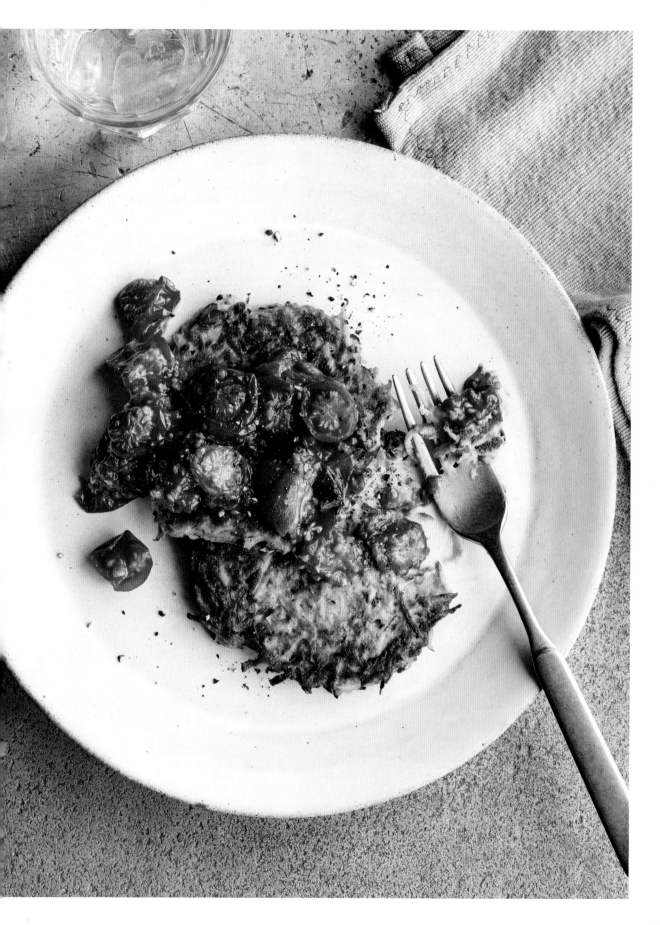

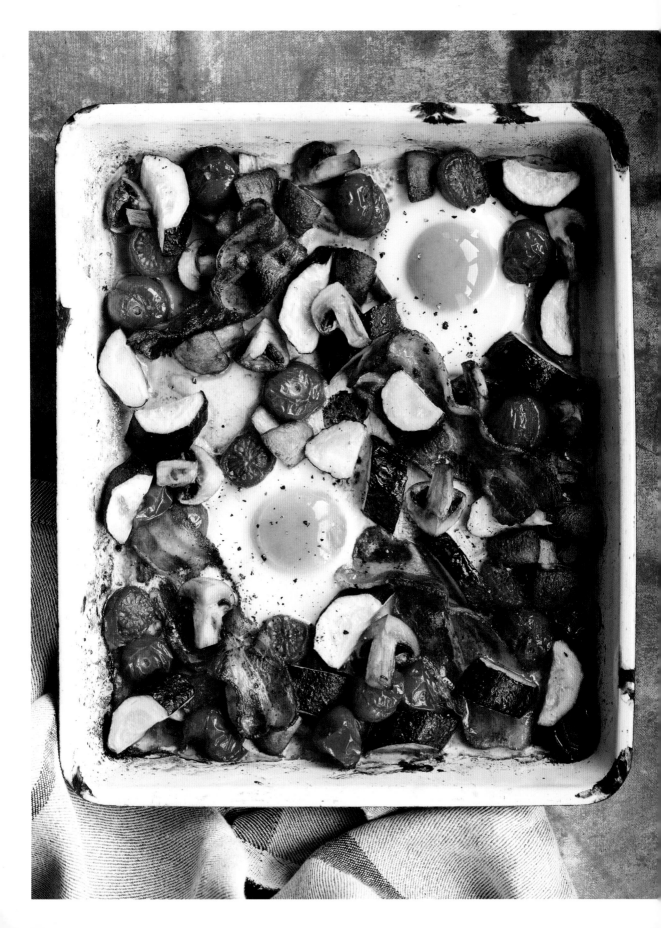

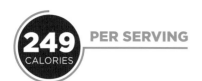

249 CALORIES **PER SERVING**

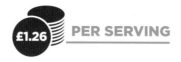

£1.26 **PER SERVING**

ONE-DISH COOKED BREAKFAST
SERVES 2

Baking the eggs in the tray with the rest of the ingredients means you use less oil – you want to create a little nest in between the vegetables and bacon so they are contained.

1 courgette, roughly
   chopped
200g mushrooms, sliced
150g cherry tomatoes,
   halved
2 tsp vegetable oil
4 rashers unsmoked
   back bacon
2 eggs
Black pepper

1 Preheat the oven to 200°C/Fan 180°C.

2 Place the courgettes, mushrooms and cherry tomatoes in a large roasting tin, drizzle with the oil, season with black pepper and roast in the oven for 20 minutes.

3 Remove the vegetables from the oven and move them to one end of the roasting tin. Lay the bacon on the other end and return to the oven for 5 minutes.

4 Finally, remove the tin from the oven once more, make some space between the bacon and vegetables, crack in the eggs and return to the oven for 8–10 minutes until the eggs are just cooked.

5 Divide the eggs, bacon and veg between two plates and serve straight away.

LUNCH

OPEN SANDWICHES THREE WAYS

Here are three ideas for lunchtime toast toppers. They're all quick to prepare and have a good balance of protein and veg to keep you going through the afternoon. They are also a low-calorie lunch option – great if you want to splurge your calorie allowance on dinner.

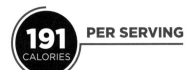 **PER SERVING**

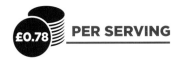 **PER SERVING**

1 TOMATO, BASIL & BUTTERBEAN
SERVES 2

175g tomatoes, diced
15g fresh basil, chopped
1 × 400g tin butterbeans, drained and roughly mashed
1 clove garlic, finely chopped
1 tbsp olive oil
2 slices rye or wholemeal bread, toasted
Black pepper

1 Combine the tomatoes with half the basil in a bowl. Season with black pepper and set aside.

2 Place the butterbeans in a separate bowl and add the garlic, olive oil and remaining basil. Season with black pepper and mix well.

3 To serve, divide the butterbean mixture between the two slices of toast and top with the tomatoes.

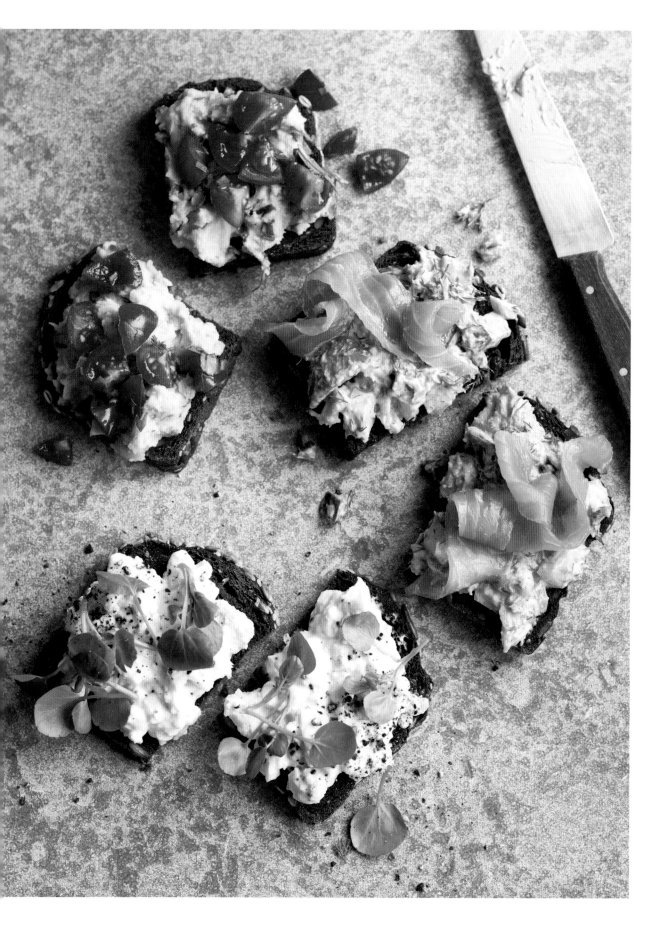

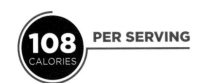

108 CALORIES — PER SERVING

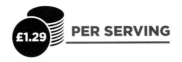

£1.29 — PER SERVING

2 CREAMY CUCUMBER & SMOKED SALMON
SERVES 2

100g cucumber, diced
½ avocado, mashed
65g natural yoghurt
10g fresh dill, chopped
Zest of ½ lemon
2 slices rye or wholemeal
   bread, toasted
75g smoked salmon, sliced
Black pepper

1 Combine the cucumber, avocado, yoghurt, dill and lemon zest in a bowl. Season with pepper, mix well and set aside.

2 To serve, divide the cucumber mixture between the two slices of toast and top with slices of smoked salmon.

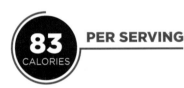

83 CALORIES — PER SERVING

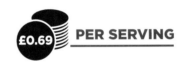

£0.69 — PER SERVING

3 EGG, COTTAGE CHEESE & ROCKET
SERVES 2

2 eggs
150g cottage cheese
2 slices rye or wholemeal
   bread, toasted
A handful of watercress,
   rocket or any salad leaves
Black pepper

1 Boil the eggs in a pan for 8 minutes then remove from the heat and leave to cool slightly in a bowl of cold water. Peel the eggs and place in a bowl with the cottage cheese. Season with black pepper and mash everything together well.

2 To serve, divide the egg mixture between the two slices of toast and top with the salad leaves.

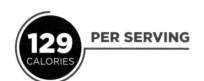

129 CALORIES **PER SERVING**

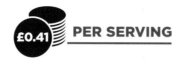

£0.41 **PER SERVING**

SUNSHINE SOUP
SERVES 4

A zesty, warming and low-calorie soup packed full of good-for-you ingredients. This soup is creamy and sweet and a great one to try on kids or soup sceptics. It will keep well in the fridge for a few days and also freezes perfectly. Freeze the soup in individual portions and defrost overnight (or in the microwave) for those days when you're short of time. Keep an eye out for frozen butternut squash chunks in your local supermarket; they are a thrifty and time-saving ingredient to have in your freezer. (See photo on page 84.)

1 tbsp olive oil
1 onion, chopped
2 cloves garlic, chopped
1 small butternut squash, deseeded and roughly chopped (no need to peel it)
3 carrots, roughly chopped
1 tsp ground turmeric
1.5l vegetable stock (fresh or made using 2 low-salt stock cubes)
Black pepper

1 Heat the oil in a saucepan over a medium heat and sauté the onion for 5 minutes until soft.

2 Add the garlic and cook for a further 2 minutes, then stir in the squash, carrots and turmeric.

3 Pour the vegetable stock into the pan and bring to a light boil. Reduce the heat and simmer for 20–30 minutes until the vegetables are nice and soft.

4 Remove from the heat and leave to cool for 10–20 minutes. Pour the soup into a food processor and whizz until smooth. Season with black pepper. Add a little more water or stock if you prefer a thinner soup.

5 Return to the pan, check the seasoning and reheat gently to serve.

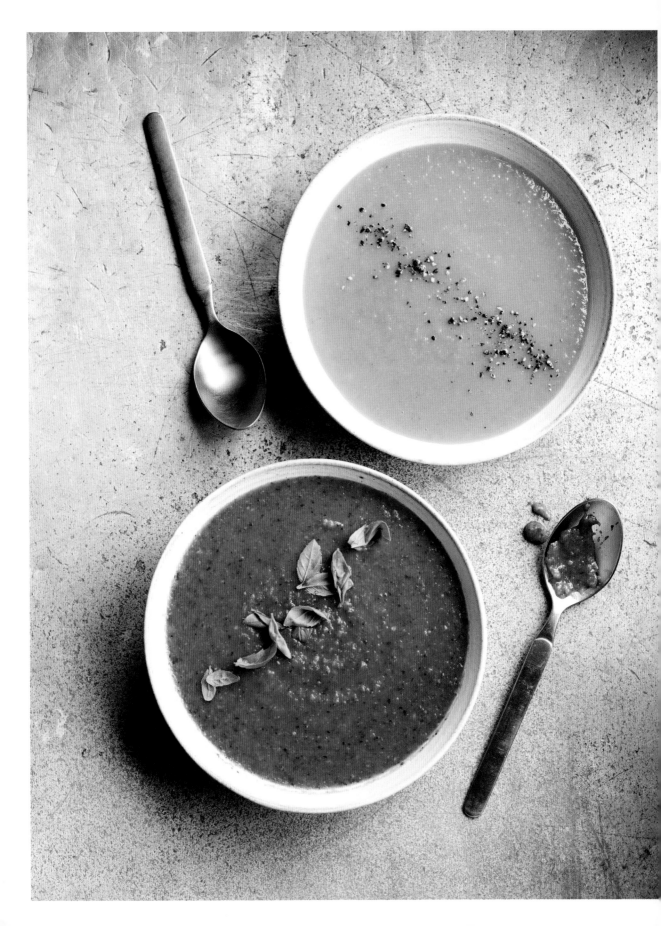

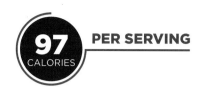

PER SERVING

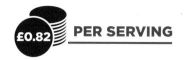

£0.82 PER SERVING

CREAMY ROAST TOMATO & BASIL SOUP
SERVES 4

This is a wonderful soup to make in the summer months when tomatoes are really flavourful and inexpensive. Roasting the tomatoes and garlic, instead of cooking them on the hob, gives an amazing depth of flavour. (Also pictured is **Sunshine Soup**, recipe on page 83.)

1kg tomatoes, halved
1 red onion, roughly
   chopped
1 carrot, roughly chopped
4 cloves garlic, peeled
   but kept whole
1 tbsp olive oil
600ml vegetable stock
   (fresh or made using
   1 low-salt stock cube)
2 tbsp natural yoghurt
15g fresh basil, plus
   extra to serve
Black pepper

1 Preheat the oven to 180°C/Fan 160°C.

2 Place the tomatoes, onion, carrot and garlic in a large roasting tray and drizzle with the olive oil. Roast in the oven for 1½ hours until everything is soft and sticky.

3 Tip the cooked vegetables and their juices into a food processor. Add the stock, yoghurt and basil, season with black pepper and whizz until smooth.

4 When you are ready to serve, pour the soup into a saucepan and place over a medium heat to warm through. Serve garnished with basil leaves.

SOUP CAN SAVE YOUR DIET!
Soup is easy to cook in bulk; it's packed with vegetables and, because of the water content, it's a high-volume, low-cost, low-calorie food that will help you to feel full. Avoid adding cream and butter.

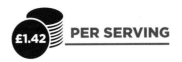
MINESTRONE WITH PESTO
SERVES 4

This is a great family meal – it's really filling and hearty but also nutritious and low cal. Use whichever vegetables you have or, if the fridge is bare, frozen peas or tinned sweetcorn also work well.

1 tbsp vegetable oil
1 onion, diced
3 carrots, diced
3 cloves garlic, finely chopped
600g tomatoes,
    roughly chopped
2l chicken or vegetable
    stock (fresh or made using
    2 low-salt stock cubes)
1 × 400g tin cannellini
    beans, drained
100g small dried pasta
    shapes (such as macaroni
    or conchigliette)
300g green vegetables
    (use what's in season,
    such as broccoli, spinach,
    chard and green beans)
Black pepper

For the pesto
30g fresh basil
30g fresh flat-leaf parsley
3 tbsp olive oil
35g unsalted almonds
1 clove garlic

1 To make the pesto, place all the ingredients in a food processor with 2 tablespoons of water and whizz until blended.

2 Heat the oil in a large casserole pan over a medium to low heat. Add the onion and carrots and cook for 15 minutes until soft.

3 Stir in the garlic and cook for another 2 minutes, stirring regularly to ensure it doesn't burn.

4 Add the tomatoes and cook for 5 minutes, stirring regularly. Pour in the stock and cannellini beans and simmer for 20 minutes.

5 Meanwhile, cook the pasta according to the packet instructions, until just cooked but al dente. Drain well and set aside.

6 Add the green vegetables to the casserole pan and cook for a further 5 minutes until soft. If you are not serving the minestrone straight away, leave the pasta out until you are ready to serve. Otherwise, tip the pasta into the pan, loosen with a little boiling water if needed, and season with black pepper.

7 Serve the soup in bowls with a drizzle of the pesto over the top.

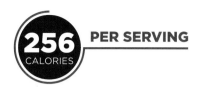
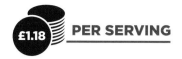
DIY INSTANT MISO VEGGIE SOUP JARS
SERVES 2

These are a really quick, low-calorie yet satisfying packed lunch to take into the office. Perfect for when you want something warming on a cold day. You can add a boiled egg or some leftover cooked chicken or fish to the jars too to boost your protein intake.

50g spinach (fresh or frozen), roughly chopped
2 tbsp miso paste
2 tbsp low-salt soy sauce
200g cooked grains (quinoa or brown rice are best)
1 carrot, grated
75g mushrooms, sliced
15g fresh soft herbs, roughly chopped (use one or a mixture of parsley, basil, coriander and dill)
Juice of ½ lemon
Pinch of chilli flakes

1 If using frozen spinach, defrost either in the microwave (place in a bowl and cook on high for 1–2 minutes) or place in a sieve over the sink and pour boiling water over the top. Squeeze and drain out the excess water.

2 Divide all of the ingredients between two jars or airtight containers.

3 When you are ready to eat, pour over 300ml of boiling water per jar and mix well. Cover with the lid or a plate and leave for 2–3 minutes before eating. You could also make this in a bowl if you are eating it straight away.

USE YOUR FREEZER
Don't let leftover fresh herbs go to waste or linger at the back of the fridge – freeze them in ice cube trays instead. Finely chop the herbs, spoon into ice cube trays, fill each hole with a little bit of water and pop in the freezer. They will keep there for months. Simply add a whole cube straight from the freezer to soups, stews, curries or sauces.

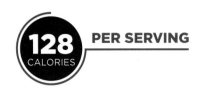

PER SERVING 128 CALORIES

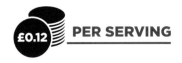

PER SERVING £0.12

HOMEMADE SPINACH WRAPS
SERVES 4

These are the perfect healthy alternative to white flour tortillas when you're in the mood for a wrap. Frozen spinach is a real wonder ingredient; it comes in a big bag in little nuggets that you can defrost one at a time – very good value for money and a quick and easy way to get extra greens in. Eat the wraps open at home or roll them up for a packed lunch. Filling ideas: roasted vegetables with Chickpea and Pesto Dip on page 190; leftover Slow-cooked Lamb on page 162 with lettuce and natural yoghurt; or mashed avocado and cooked chicken.

85g frozen spinach
65g plain flour
1 egg
150ml semi-skimmed milk
1 tbsp vegetable oil

1 Defrost the spinach – either in the microwave (place in a bowl and cook on high for 1–2 minutes) or place in a sieve over the sink and pour boiling water over the top. Squeeze and drain out the excess water.

2 Place the flour, egg, milk and spinach in a food processor and whizz until you have a smooth batter.

3 Heat a little of the oil in a large non-stick frying pan over a medium heat. Add a ladleful of the spinach mixture, swirling it around the pan to coat, and cook for 1 minute on each side, or until golden. Repeat with the remaining mixture to make three more wraps.

4 Serve straight away or save to eat later. The wraps freeze very well between baking parchment.

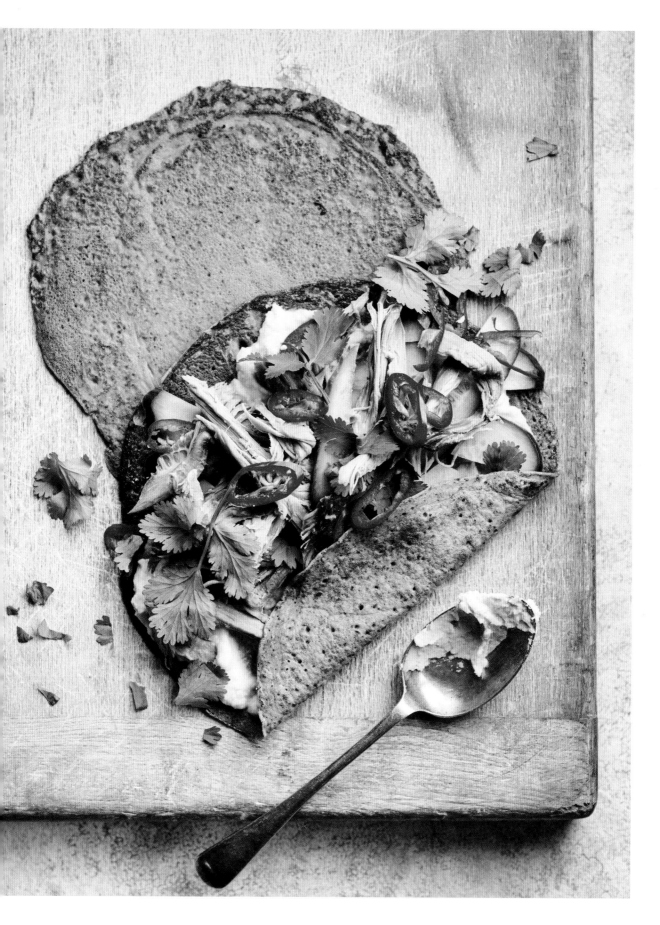

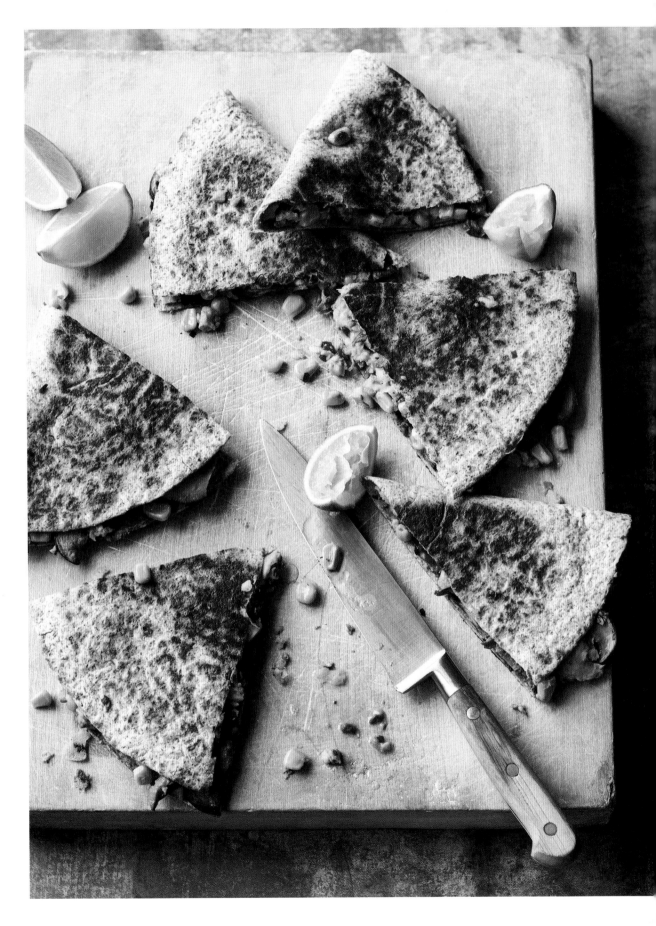

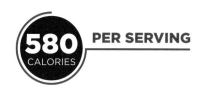
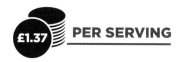
CHEESY MUSHROOM, AVOCADO & SWEETCORN QUESADILLA
SERVES 4

This is basically a Mexican cheese toastie, with more flavour than the British variety! It's a crowd pleaser and really popular with kids, too – just leave out the chilli if they're little.

1 tbsp vegetable oil
300g mushrooms, sliced
4 cloves garlic,
   finely chopped
1 red chilli, finely chopped
4 wholemeal tortilla wraps
100g Cheddar, grated
2 × 198g tins low-salt
   sweetcorn, drained
2 avocados, mashed
30g fresh coriander,
   chopped
1 lime, cut into wedges,
   to serve
Black pepper

1 Heat the oil in a frying pan over a medium heat, add the mushrooms and cook for 10 minutes until golden brown. Add the garlic and chilli and cook for a further few minutes, stirring regularly to ensure it doesn't burn. Tip the garlic and chilli mushrooms out of the frying pan and into a bowl. Season with black pepper and set aside.

2 To assemble the quesadillas, lay a wrap on a plate or board and sprinkle some cheese over the bottom half. Top this with a quarter of the mushroom mixture and a quarter of the sweetcorn, followed by a quarter of the mashed avocado. Sprinkle with a little more cheese and a quarter of the coriander then fold the wrap in half.

3 Place a non-stick frying pan over a medium heat. Add the folded wrap to the pan and cook for 2–3 minutes on each side. As it cooks, press down quite firmly with a spatula or place a plate on top. When both sides are toasted and the cheese has melted, remove from the pan. Repeat with the other wraps.

4 Serve the quesadillas with a wedge of fresh lime.

 **PER SERVING**

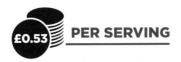 **PER SERVING**

NEW POTATO & COURGETTE FRITTATA
SERVES 4

A one pan, quick and easy lunch that also keeps well for a packed lunch the next day – just slice the frittata up into portions and keep them in an airtight container in the fridge. It's a great low-calorie and low-cost meal for all the family.

350g new potatoes, roughly chopped
2 tsp unsalted butter
1 onion, sliced
1 courgette, diced
6 eggs, beaten
15g fresh flat-leaf parsley, chopped
Black pepper

1 Boil the potatoes in a pan of water for 5 minutes, or until just tender. Drain and set aside.

2 Meanwhile, heat the butter in a non-stick frying pan over a low heat. Add the onion and sauté for 10 minutes until soft. Turn the heat up, add the courgette and cooked potato and cook for 2–3 minutes, until the potato and courgette are starting to brown.

3 Pour the eggs into the pan, sprinkle the parsley over the top and season with black pepper. Give it a quick stir to ensure the vegetables are all encased within the egg, pulling the egg in from the sides. Leave to cook for 2–3 minutes until it is starting to set. Finally, place it under the grill for 2 minutes to cook the top or slide the frittata on to a plate and flip it over back into the pan to cook the other side for a further minute.

4 Serve with a simple green salad.

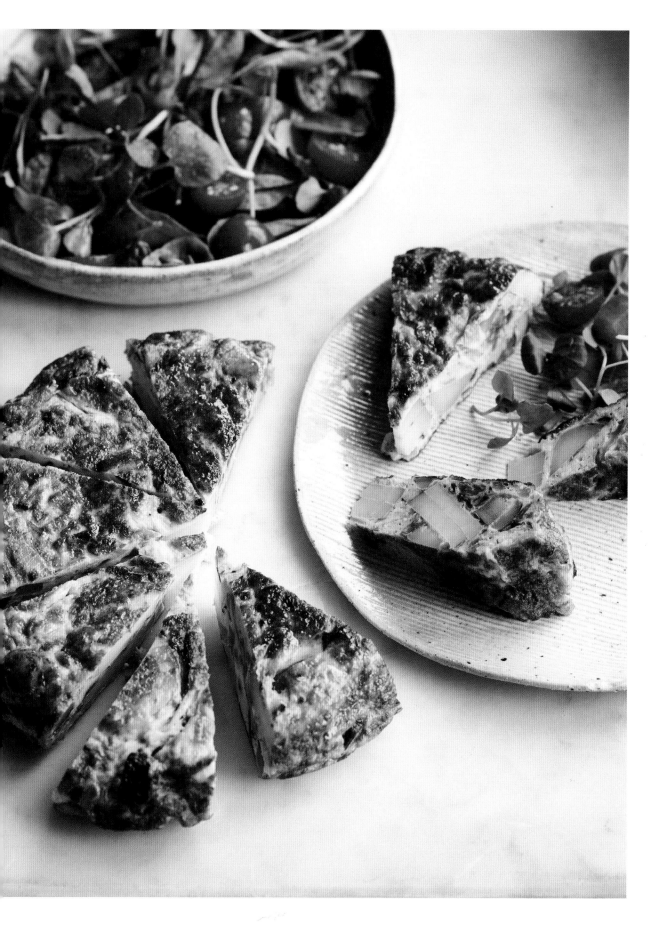

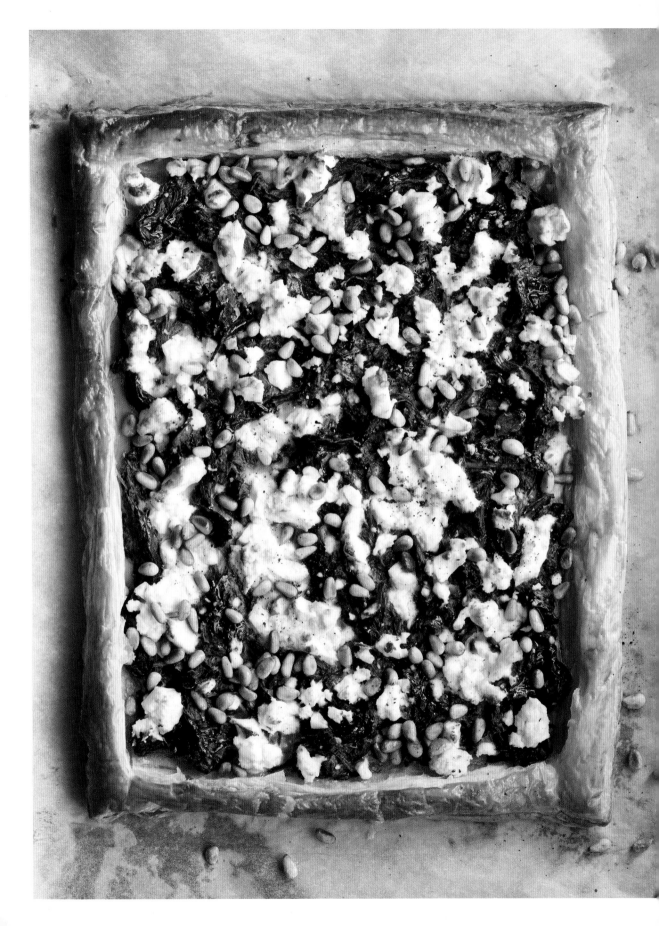

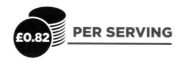
SPINACH & FETA TART
SERVES 4

This tart is quick, easy and really delicious and, most importantly, it doesn't feel like diet food. It's a great recipe for entertaining – any leftovers taste great eaten cold the next day! Serves four as a main meal or six as a lighter lunch.

300g frozen spinach
3 eggs, beaten
¼ nutmeg, grated
1 × 320g packet ready-rolled
    puff pastry
150g feta, crumbled
25g pine nuts
Black pepper

1 Preheat the oven to 200°C/Fan 180°C and line a baking tray with baking parchment.

2 Defrost the spinach – either in the microwave (place in a bowl and cook on high for 1–2 minutes) or place in a sieve over the sink and pour boiling water over the top. Drain and squeeze out any excess water and add the spinach to a bowl. Add the eggs and nutmeg to the bowl and season with pepper. Stir to combine.

3 Unroll the puff pastry and place on the prepared baking tray. Using a sharp knife, score a rectangle approximately 3cm inside the edges of the pastry, making sure you don't cut through the pastry. Place in the oven and bake blind for 10 minutes.

4 Remove the pastry from the oven and spoon the spinach and egg mixture into the centre, spreading it out evenly to the edges of the scored rectangle. Sprinkle the feta and pine nuts over the top and bake in the oven for 20 minutes until golden brown.

5 Serve the tart with a salad of green leaves.

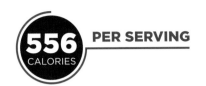
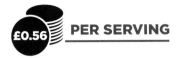

RAINBOW VEGETABLE & FETA SALAD

SERVES 2

A satisfying yet healthy salad that can be made the day before as it keeps really well for a packed lunch. You can mix up the vegetables and use up whatever you have in the fridge.

160g couscous
1 tbsp olive oil
1 tbsp balsamic vinegar
½ clove garlic, finely
    chopped
1 large carrot, coarsely
    grated
2 small cooked beetroot,
    cut into chunks
½ cucumber, diced
2 spring onions, finely sliced
100g feta, crumbled
Pinch of chilli flakes
    (optional)
Black pepper

1 Measure the couscous into a heatproof serving bowl and just cover with 250ml boiling water. Cover the bowl with a plate and leave for 10 minutes.

2 Whisk the olive oil and balsamic vinegar together in a small bowl or pour them into a jam jar and give it a good shake. Season with black pepper and add the garlic. Mix or shake again.

3 Fluff the couscous with a fork then stir in the veg and dressing. Crumble in the feta and sprinkle with chilli flakes, if using, to serve.

COLOUR

Make your plate as colourful as you can because brightly coloured fruit and vegetables will do wonders for your health and waistline.

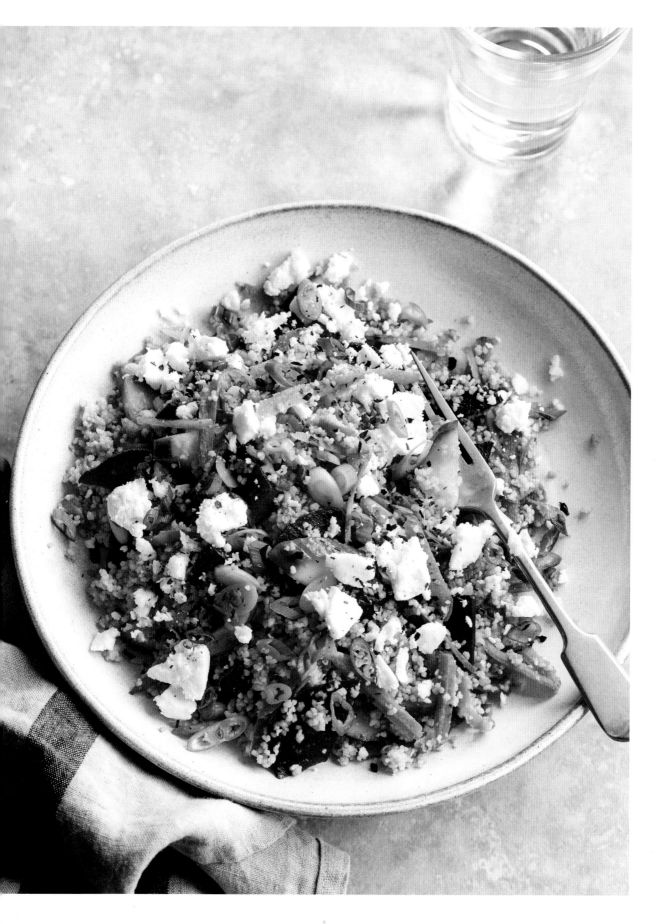

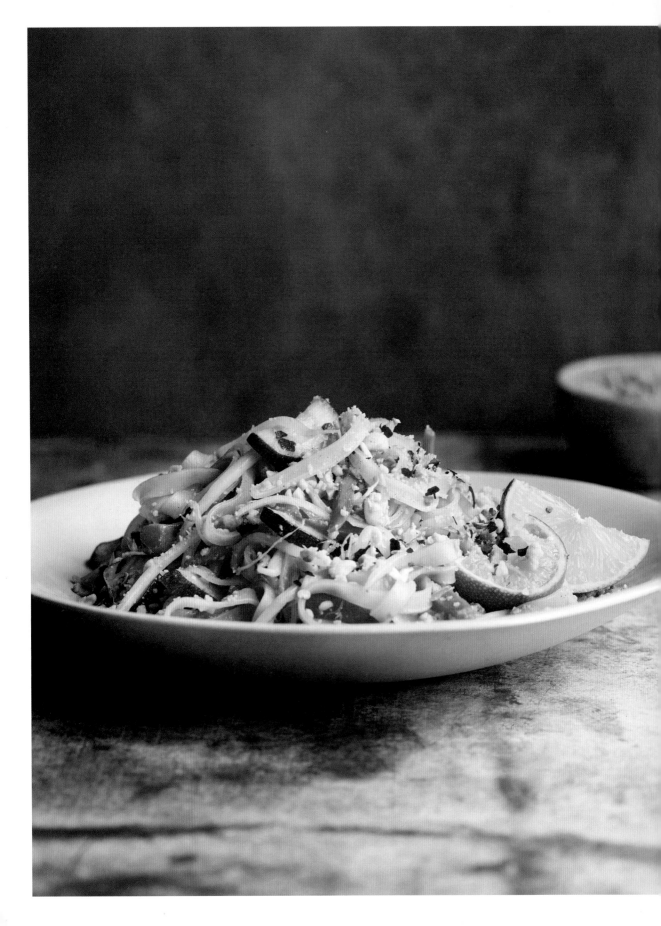

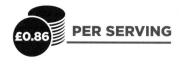

VEGETABLE PAD THAI
SERVES 4

A simple version of the takeaway favourite that won't blow the calories or the budget. It's great for the whole family, is crammed full of veggies and includes lots of protein from the eggs and nuts.

200g rice noodles
1 tbsp vegetable oil
2 carrots, grated or
    peeled into ribbons
2 courgettes, sliced into
    half moons
200g beansprouts
3 cloves garlic, finely
    chopped
4 tbsp low-salt soy sauce
2 tbsp honey
4 tsp fish sauce
Pinch of chilli flakes, plus
    extra to serve (optional)
4 tsp cornflour
2 eggs, beaten
35g unsalted peanuts,
    chopped
Lime wedges, to serve

1 Cook the noodles according to the packet instructions. Drain, rinse with cold water and set aside.

2 Heat the oil in a large frying pan over a high heat. Add the carrot, courgette and beansprouts to the pan and sauté for 1–2 minutes until starting to soften. Add the garlic and cook for a further 1–2 minutes, stirring regularly to ensure it doesn't burn.

3 Meanwhile, in a small bowl or mug, mix together the soy sauce, honey, fish sauce, chilli flakes and cornflour. Add this mixture to the pan and cook for 1 minute. Move the vegetable mixture to one side of the pan, pour in the egg and leave to set before scrambling it and mixing with the vegetables.

4 Finally, add the noodles, stir to combine everything and cook until hot through.

5 Sprinkle with the chopped peanuts and chilli flakes, if using, and serve with lime wedges.

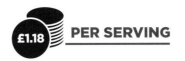

RAINBOW VEG STUFFED SWEET POTATOES
SERVES 4

A jazzed-up jacket potato but with loads of good-for-you ingredients. You can make these ahead of time and reheat them in a low oven. The vegetables are also interchangeable here – use what you have in the fridge, just make sure you chop everything finely. The quinoa is a great plant-based source of protein.

4 sweet potatoes
2 tbsp vegetable oil
200g quinoa
1 bunch of spring onions, sliced
2 courgettes, diced
2 red peppers, diced
2 carrots, diced
2 cloves garlic, finely chopped
2 tsp ground coriander
Black pepper

1 Preheat the oven to 200°C/Fan 180°C.

2 Slice the sweet potatoes in half lengthways, place them on a roasting tin and brush with 1 tablespoon of the oil. Bake in the oven for 40 minutes, until soft.

3 Meanwhile, cook the quinoa according to the packet instructions. Drain and set aside.

4 Heat the remaining oil in a large pan over a medium heat. Add the spring onions, courgettes, red peppers and carrots, and cook for 10 minutes until the vegetables are soft.

5 Add the garlic and ground coriander and cook for a further 5 minutes, stirring regularly to ensure it doesn't burn. Scoop out the flesh of the sweet potatoes (keeping the skins intact) and place in a large bowl with the cooked vegetables and quinoa. Season with black pepper and combine well.

6 Spoon the vegetable mixture back into the sweet potato skins and serve.

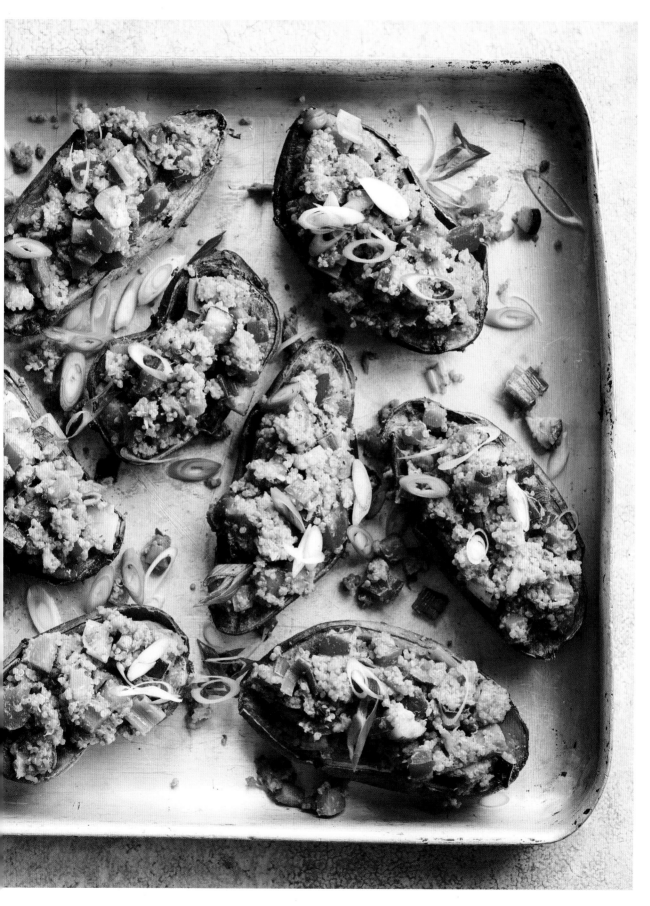

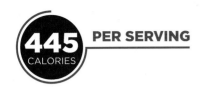

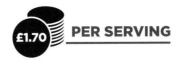

SPICED ROAST CHICKPEA & CAULIFLOWER SALAD
SERVES 2

This is a great, alternative way to serve cauliflower. It is very nice served warm but equally delicious cold, so would make a lovely packed lunch. Just remember to dress it at the last minute so the salad leaves don't go soggy. This is also a good side dish to jazz up some simple grilled fish or meat.

2 tbsp vegetable oil
2 tsp smoked paprika
1 tsp ground cumin
2 tsp ground turmeric
1 small cauliflower (approx. 400g), cut into small florets
1 × 400g tin chickpeas, drained
125g salad leaves
Black pepper

For the dressing
1 tbsp olive oil
2 tbsp cider vinegar
Pinch of chilli flakes
1 tsp honey
1 clove garlic, finely chopped
15g fresh coriander, finely chopped
15g fresh flat-leaf parsley, finely chopped

1 Preheat the oven to 220°C/Fan 200°C.

2 In a small bowl, mix together the vegetable oil, paprika, cumin and turmeric with some black pepper to make a paste.

3 Place the cauliflower and drained chickpeas in a roasting tray and spoon over the spiced paste. Mix everything together well with your hands so the cauliflower and chickpeas are well coated. Place in the oven and roast for 25 minutes, giving them a quick stir halfway through the cooking time to ensure they roast evenly.

4 Meanwhile, mix all of the dressing ingredients together in a mug or small bowl with 2 tablespoons of water.

5 To assemble the salad, place the salad leaves in a large serving dish and top with the roasted cauliflower and chickpeas. Drizzle with the dressing to serve.

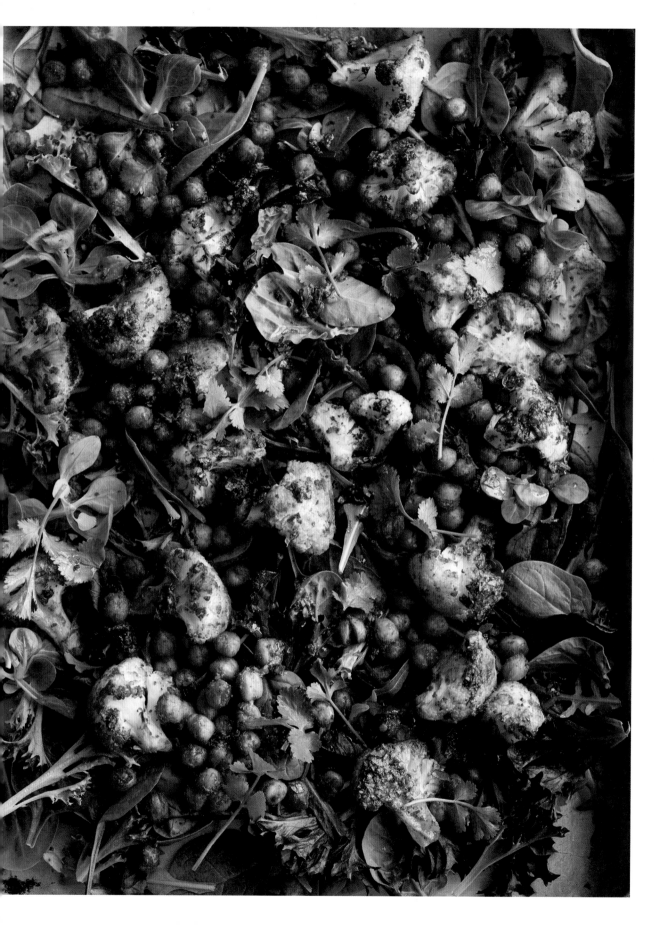

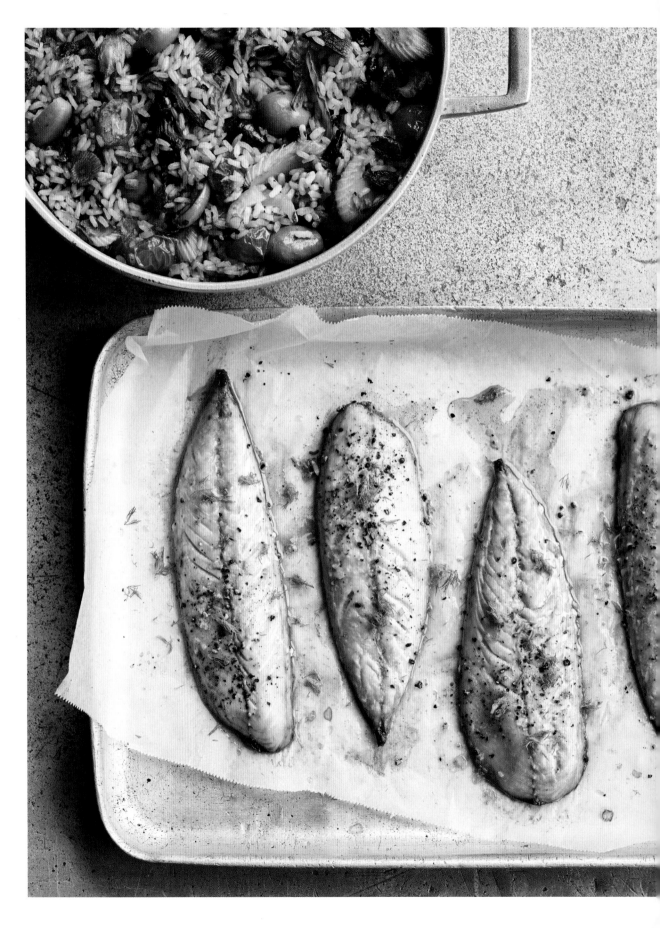

388 CALORIES **PER SERVING**

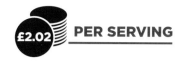

£2.02 **PER SERVING**

MEDITERRANEAN MACKEREL & BAKED RICE
SERVES 4

Mackerel is often overlooked but it's a great fish packed with good fats, is really cheap compared to a lot of other fresh fish and is easy to cook. Baking the rice means all the lovely flavours of the stock and vegetables are soaked into the rice while it cooks.

1 tbsp vegetable oil
1 red onion, chopped
1 bulb of fennel, finely sliced, reserving some fronds to garnish
4 cloves garlic, finely chopped
250g cherry tomatoes
180g black or green olives, pitted and halved
175g brown basmati rice
2 tsp balsamic vinegar
Zest and juice of 1 lemon
400ml chicken stock (fresh or made using 1 low-salt stock cube)
4 mackerel fillets
1 tbsp olive oil
Black pepper

1 Preheat the oven to 200°C/Fan 180°C and line a baking tray with baking parchment.

2 Place the vegetable oil in an ovenproof, heavy-based pan that has a lid over a medium heat. Add the onion and fennel and sauté for 10 minutes, until soft.

3 Turn down the heat, add the garlic, tomatoes and olives and cook for a further 5 minutes, stirring regularly so the garlic doesn't burn.

4 Add the rice, balsamic vinegar, lemon zest and juice and the stock, cover with the lid, place in the oven and cook for 1 hour.

5 Twenty minutes before the end of the cooking time, place the mackerel on the prepared baking tray, drizzle with the olive oil, season with black pepper and place in the oven with the vegetables and rice for 20 minutes.

6 Remove both dishes from the oven and serve with the reserved fennel fronds sprinkled over the mackerel.

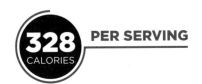
PER SERVING

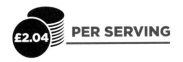
PER SERVING

ZINGY PRAWN & NOODLE SALAD JAR SHAKERS
SERVES 2

These flavour-packed salad jars are low calorie but the generous portions will fill you up. Perfect to make the night before, just pour the dressing over when you're ready to eat and give the jar a good shake.

1 × 60g nest dried
  egg noodles
150g cooked king prawns
1 carrot, grated or
  finely sliced
½ cucumber, grated
  or finely sliced
2 Little Gem lettuces,
  roughly chopped
15g fresh coriander,
  roughly chopped

For the dressing
Zest and juice of 1 lime
½ clove garlic, finely
  chopped
2 tbsp low-salt soy sauce
2 tbsp olive oil
2 tsp honey
Black pepper

1 Cook the noodles according to the packet instructions. Drain, rinse in cold water and set aside.

2 Divide the prawns, cooked noodles, carrot, cucumber, Little Gems and coriander between two jars or pots.

3 In a separate container, mix together all of the dressing ingredients.

4 When you're ready to eat the salads, pour the dressing into the jars, shake them up and serve!

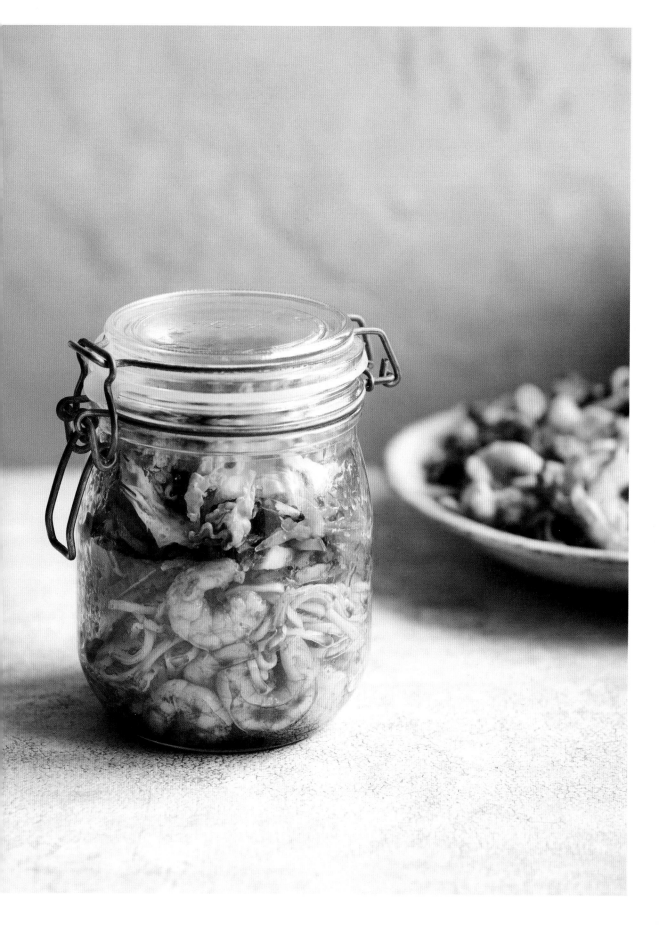

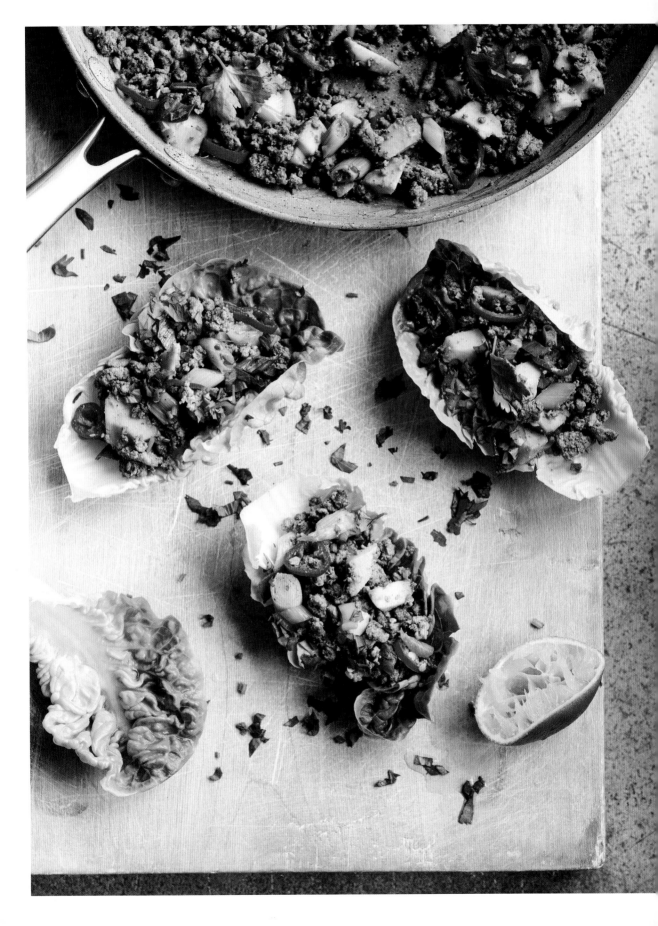

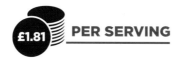
SPICED TURKEY MINCE & AVOCADO LETTUCE CUPS
SERVES 4

This is a fun and easy way to put a dish together. Turkey mince is a good low-calorie swap for beef or pork mince and it's great value, too. Kids will love these – just skip the chilli for theirs.

1 tbsp vegetable oil
500g turkey mince
3 cloves garlic, finely chopped
2 tsp Chinese 5 spice
2 tbsp low-salt soy sauce
2 avocados, diced
1 bunch of spring onions, sliced
1 red chilli, sliced
Juice of 1 lime
4 Little Gem lettuces, separated into leaves (keep the smaller inside leaves for a salad)
15g fresh coriander, chopped

1 Heat the oil in a non-stick frying pan over a high heat. Add the turkey mince and cook for 5 minutes until starting to brown. Lower the heat, add the garlic and Chinese 5 spice and sauté for a further 5 minutes. Add the soy sauce and 3 tablespoons of water and leave to simmer for 10 minutes.

2 Finally, add the avocado, spring onions, chilli and lime juice, and stir everything together well.

3 Spoon the turkey mixture into the Little Gem leaves and sprinkle with the coriander to serve.

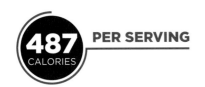 **PER SERVING**

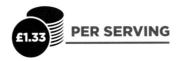 **PER SERVING**

487 CALORIES

£1.33

ASIAN CHICKEN SALAD
SERVES 2

Full of vibrant flavours and perfect for using up leftover roast chicken, you can play with the protein here, too, as this would work well with salmon, smoked mackerel or prawns.

1 skinless and boneless chicken breast (or 150g leftover/cooked chicken)
1 low-salt chicken stock cube (if using raw chicken)
75g rice noodles
¼ red cabbage, thinly sliced
2 carrots, grated or peeled into ribbons
100g sugar snap peas, sliced lengthways
15g fresh herbs, chopped (e.g. coriander, mint or basil or a combination)

For the dressing
25g peanut butter
1 tbsp sesame oil
1 tbsp honey
Juice of 1 lime
1 tbsp white wine vinegar

1 If using raw chicken, bring a small pan of water to the boil, add the stock cube and the chicken breast and simmer for 10–15 minutes over a low heat until the chicken breast is cooked through. Drain and set aside to cool.

2 Cook the noodles according to the packet instructions. Drain, rinse with cold water and set aside.

3 Make the dressing by whisking all of the ingredients together with a fork.

4 To assemble your salad, shred or slice the cooked chicken breast and place this in a bowl with the remaining salad ingredients. Toss to combine. Drizzle the dressing over the top and serve.

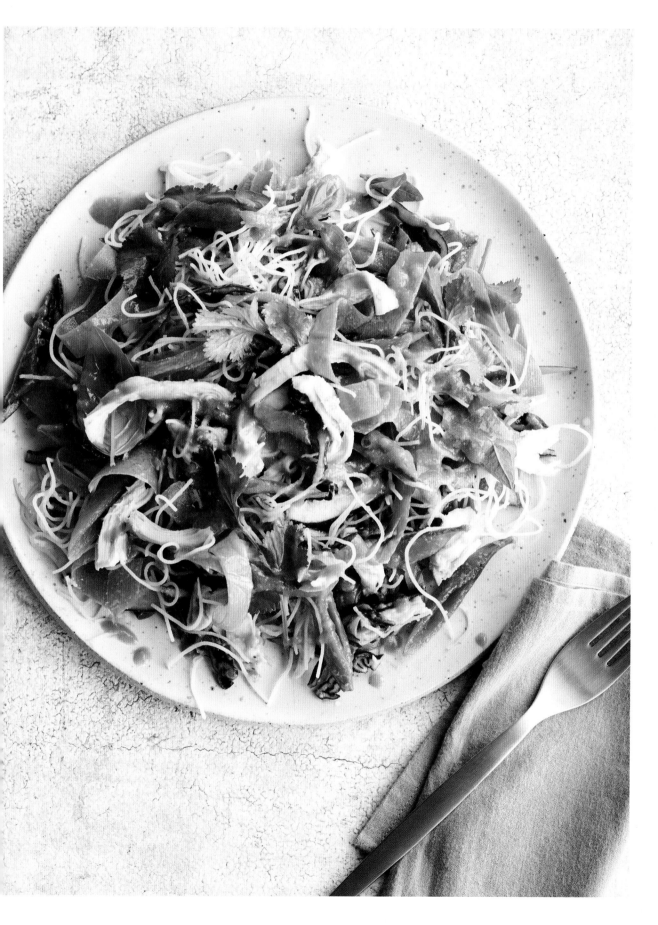

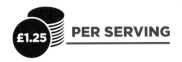

515 CALORIES **PER SERVING**

£1.25 **PER SERVING**

EASY SUNDAY ROAST CHICKEN WITH ONE-TRAY VEGETABLES
SERVES 4

A Sunday roast minus the fuss. Keep the chicken carcass to make stock – simmer for a couple of hours in a large pan of boiling water with an onion and carrot, strain and use for soup or stews, or freeze.

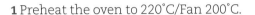

1 whole chicken
  (approx. 1.5kg)
2 tbsp vegetable oil
1 lemon
500g sweet potato, peeled
  and cut into chunks
2 onions, cut into wedges
350g carrots, cut
  into chunks
350g parsnips, peeled
  and cut into chunks
Black pepper

CHICKEN STOCK
Don't throw away your chicken carcass – place it in a large pan with an onion, a couple of carrots, some celery and peppercorns and cover with water. Bring the pan to a boil then simmer for at least an hour (the longer the better – you might need to top up the water). Strain, discarding the carcass and vegetables. You can then keep this stock in the fridge for 2–3 days or freeze.

1 Preheat the oven to 220°C/Fan 200°C.

2 Place the chicken in a large roasting tin. Drizzle 1 tablespoon of the oil over the chicken and rub it over the skin. Prick the skin of the lemon with the tip of a knife, cut it in half and insert it inside the cavity of the chicken. Season the chicken with black pepper and place in the oven to roast for 25 minutes.

3 Meanwhile, mix the sweet potato, onions, carrots and parsnip with the remaining 1 tablespoon of oil and season with black pepper.

4 Remove the chicken from the oven, lift it out of the tin and set aside. Tip the vegetables into the roasting tin and place the chicken on top of them. Return to the oven and roast the chicken and vegetables for a further 45 minutes, or until the chicken is cooked and the vegetables are tender.

5 Remove from the oven, place a large piece of foil over the chicken and vegetables and leave to rest for 10–15 minutes.

6 Serve the roast chicken and vegetables with steamed greens.

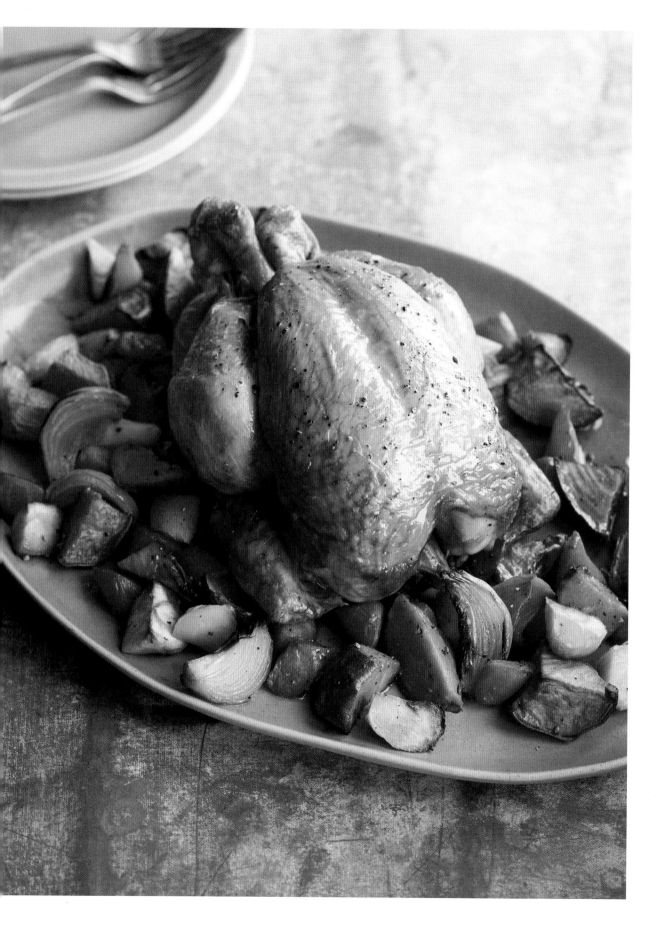

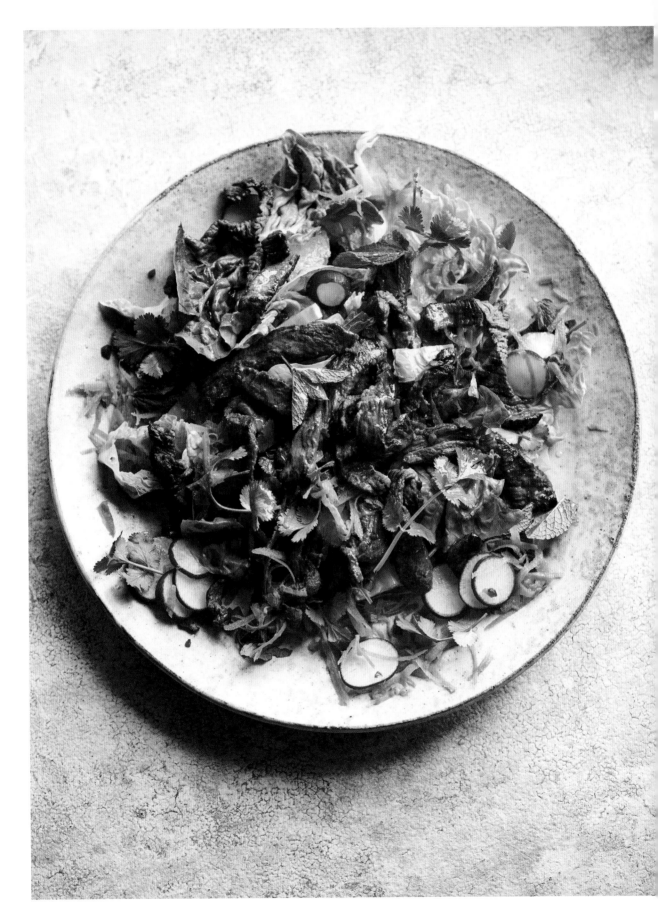

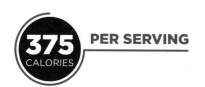
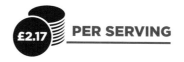
VIETNAMESE BEEF SALAD
SERVES 2

This is a quick and easy meal for when time is short and you don't want to do much cooking. Jam-packed full of flavour, the dressing and marinade add an amazing sweet and sour kick that really pulls the dish together.

180g rump steak,
  cut into thin strips

For the beef marinade
1 tbsp vegetable oil
3 cloves garlic, finely
  chopped
1 tsp fish sauce
1 tbsp honey

For the salad
1 Little Gem lettuce, sliced
2 carrots, grated
200g radishes, thinly sliced
15g fresh coriander,
  leaves picked
15g fresh mint,
  leaves picked
1 red chilli, finely chopped

For the dressing
1 tbsp sesame oil
Juice of 1 lime
2 tsp honey
Black pepper

1 For the marinade, mix all of the ingredients together in a bowl. Add the strips of beef and mix to ensure each piece is well coated. Cover and leave to marinate (ideally for a few hours but if you're short on time you can leave it for 10–15 minutes, while you prepare the rest of the salad).

2 Combine the Little Gem, carrots, radishes, coriander, mint and red chilli in a large serving bowl.

3 Make the dressing by mixing all of the ingredients together in a small bowl or jug.

4 Heat a large non-stick frying pan over a high heat and add the marinated beef. Stir-fry for 2–3 minutes (or slightly longer if you prefer the steak well cooked).

5 Tip the beef on to the salad, pour over the dressing and serve.

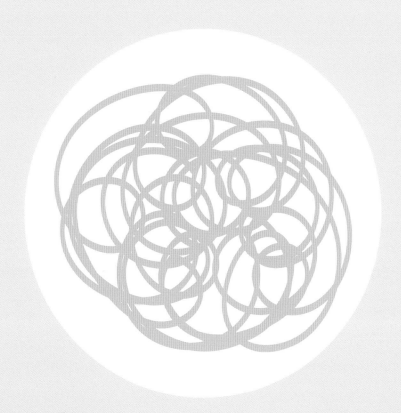

DINNER

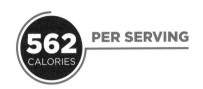
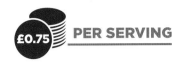
EASY HOMEMADE PIZZA
SERVES 4

Everyone loves pizza, and being able to eat it when you are trying to lose weight feels like a real treat. The base is really quick and easy to make and doesn't require any proving time. Top these with loads of veggies to keep them low calorie.

300g plain flour
1 tsp baking powder
300g natural yoghurt
400g tomato passata
1 clove garlic, crushed
Toppings of your choice,
   e.g. sliced mushrooms,
   courgette ribbons, pesto,
   cherry tomatoes, ham
2 × 125g balls mozzarella
1 tbsp olive oil
Black pepper

DITCH THE VEG DRAWER
Your veg drawer is often at the bottom of the fridge and it is very easy to lose track of what's in there. Move your veg to an eye-level shelf – you'll eat more and waste less.

1 Heat the oven to 220°C/Fan 200°C and line four baking trays with baking parchment.

2 Combine the flour, baking powder and yoghurt together in a bowl until you have a dough. Divide into four and roll out each piece on a floured worktop into a thin, round pizza base, about 20cm in diameter.

3 Meanwhile, place the passata and crushed garlic in a small pan over a medium heat and season well with black pepper. Bring to a light simmer and cook for 10 minutes. Set aside.

4 Place the pizza bases on the prepared baking trays and bake in the oven for 3 minutes until they start to puff up slightly.

5 Remove the bases from the oven, flip them over then spread the passata mixture evenly over each one. Top the pizzas with your favourite toppings, tear the mozzarella and scatter over the top, drizzle with olive oil and return them to the oven for 15 minutes, until golden brown.

6 Serve the pizzas with a green salad.

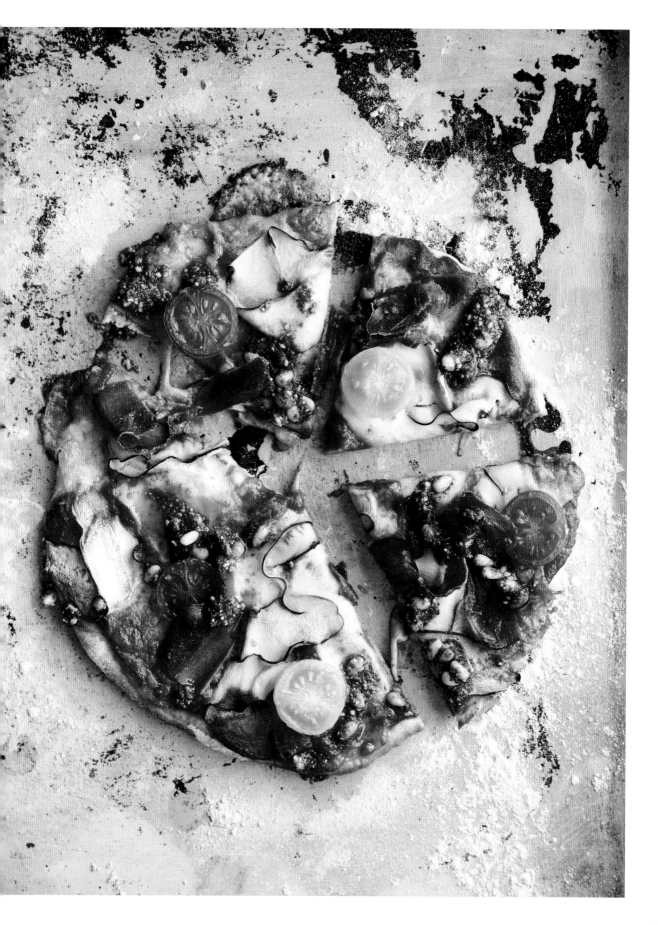

531 CALORIES · **PER SERVING**

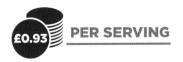
£0.93 · **PER SERVING**

SWEET POTATO GNOCCHI WITH PESTO

SERVES 4

You can prepare both the sweet potato gnocchi and the pesto sauce earlier in the day or the day before (and keep them in the fridge) – just cook the gnocchi when you're ready.

For the gnocchi
3 sweet potatoes
   (approx. 250g each)
225g plain flour (gluten-free
   also works well here)
15g cornflour

For the pesto
75g kale
30g fresh basil
6 tbsp olive oil
½ clove garlic
50g unsalted almonds
Juice of ½ lemon
2 tbsp natural yoghurt
Black pepper

WASTE NOTHING!
Don't throw away your salt-free vegetable cooking water – use it for gravies or soups instead.

1 Preheat the oven to 200°C/Fan 180°C.

2 Prick the sweet potatoes with a fork, place on a roasting tray and bake for 1 hour until soft. Leave to cool a little, then cut in half and scoop out the flesh. Measure 450g of the cooked sweet potato into a bowl and combine with the flour and cornflour. Mix to form a sticky dough, then tip out on to a lightly floured worktop and cut into four pieces. Roll each one into a sausage shape about 2cm thick and cut into 2cm slices. Press each slice slightly with a fork to flatten and set aside while you make the pesto.

3 Cook the kale in a large pan of boiling water for 2–3 minutes then drain well. Place in a food processor with 125ml water and the remaining pesto ingredients and whizz until smooth.

4 To cook the gnocchi, bring a large pan of water to the boil. Drop the gnocchi into the water and cook for 2–3 minutes, until they start to rise to the surface. You may need to do this in batches. If you overcrowd the pan, they might stick together. Drain the gnocchi, then tip back into the empty pan, add the pesto and stir to coat everything well.

5 Serve with a tomato salad or steamed vegetables.

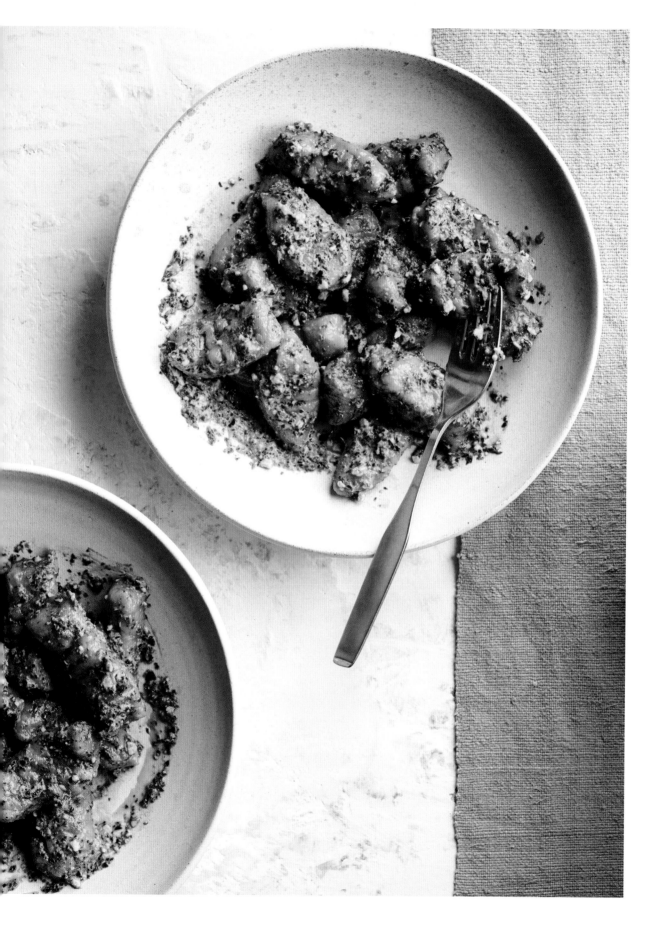

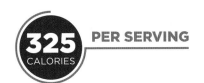
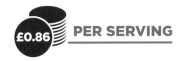

SWEET POTATO, CHICKPEA & SPINACH CURRY
SERVES 4

This is a quick and easy curry using lots of store cupboard ingredients. The base of the recipes is really versatile, meaning you can swap the vegetables and chickpeas for any other meat, pulses or vegetables.

300g brown rice
1 tbsp vegetable oil
1 onion, roughly chopped
3 cloves garlic,
    finely chopped
½–1 red chilli, finely
    chopped (optional)
3 heaped tsp garam masala
2 heaped tsp ground
    turmeric
1 × 400g tin chopped
    tomatoes
1 × 400ml tin coconut milk
2 sweet potatoes, peeled
    and diced
200ml water or any stock
1 × 400g tin chickpeas,
    drained
200g fresh spinach
    (you could use frozen)
1 tsp honey
Juice of 1 lime
Black pepper

1 Cook the rice according to the packet instructions.

2 Meanwhile, heat the oil in a large pan over a medium heat. Add the onion and sauté for 5 minutes until soft. Next, add the garlic, chilli and spices and cook for a further few minutes, stirring regularly to ensure the spices don't catch.

3 Add the chopped tomatoes, coconut milk and sweet potatoes to the pan with the water or stock. Bring to a gentle simmer and continue to cook for 15 minutes. Stir in the chickpeas and simmer for a further 15 minutes until the sweet potato is cooked.

4 Finally, add the spinach to the pan, put the lid on and turn the heat right down. After 2 minutes the spinach should be wilted enough for you to stir through the sauce with the honey and lime juice.

5 Season with black pepper and serve with the brown rice or steamed greens, depending on your calorie allowance.

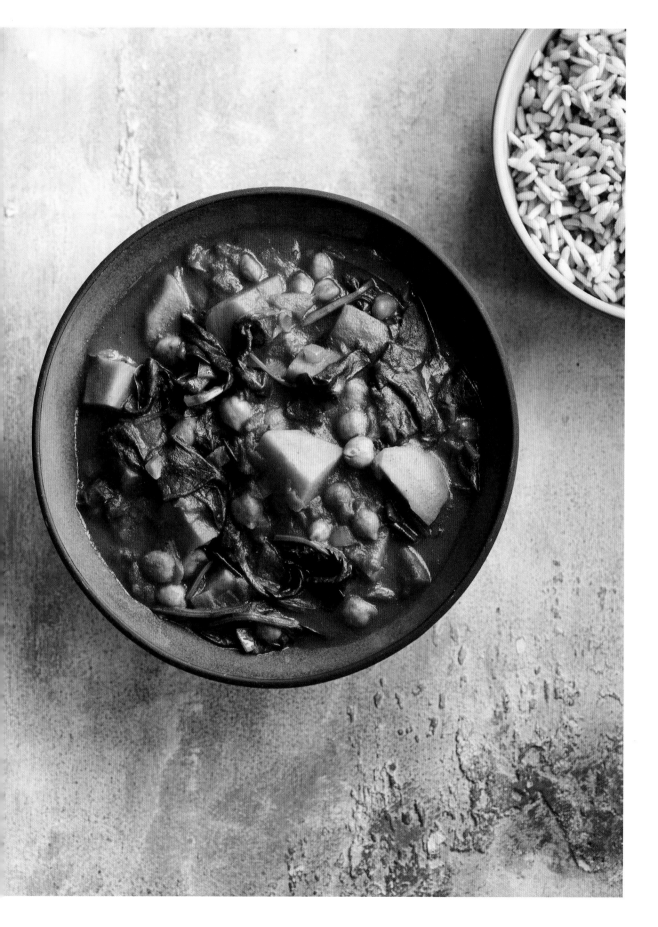

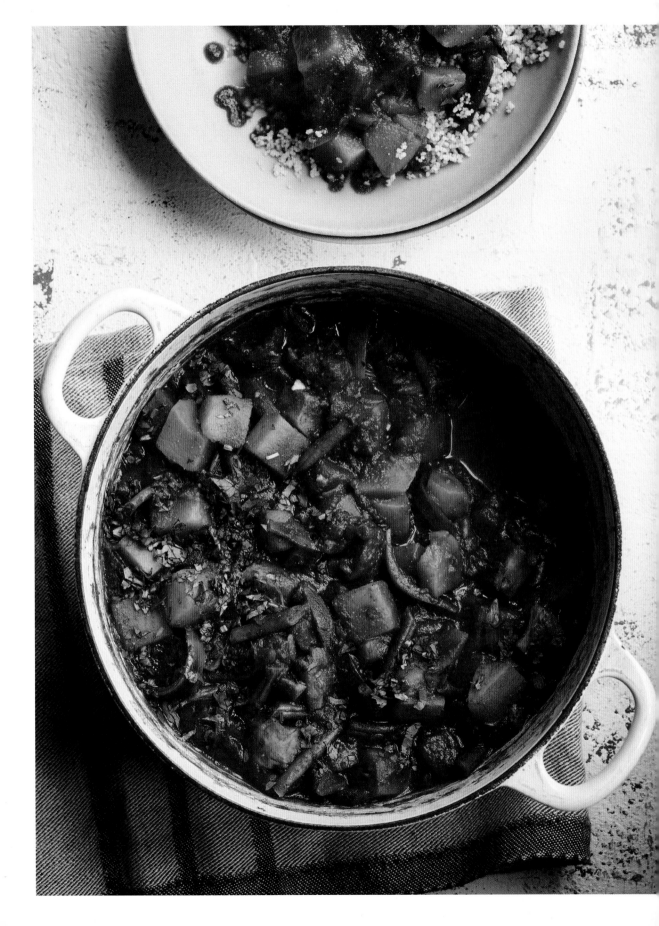

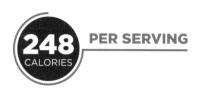
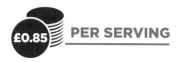

£0.85 **PER SERVING**

BUTTERNUT SQUASH & GREEN BEAN TAGINE
SERVES 4

This fragrant, hearty, vegetarian tagine has a great depth of flavour but is also really quick and easy to make. You can buy bags of peeled and chopped frozen butternut squash, which makes this dish even easier.

250g brown rice
  or couscous
1 tbsp vegetable oil
1 red onion, sliced
2 cloves garlic, finely
  chopped
2 tsp ground cinnamon
2 tsp ground cumin
2 tsp ground coriander
500g butternut squash,
  peeled and cubed
  (you can buy this frozen
  in cubes – very cheaply)
2 × 400g tins chopped
  tomatoes
140g green beans,
  roughly chopped
15g fresh coriander,
  finely chopped
Black pepper

1 Cook the rice or couscous according to the packet instructions.

2 Meanwhile, heat the oil in a heavy-based saucepan over a medium heat and sauté the onion for 10 minutes until soft.

3 Add the garlic, cinnamon, cumin and ground coriander and cook for 2 minutes, stirring so the spices don't catch.

4 Stir in the squash, tinned tomatoes and 200ml water, and leave to simmer for 15 minutes until the squash is cooked (or 25 minutes if using frozen squash).

5 Add the green beans and cook for another few minutes.

6 Finally, season with black pepper, scatter over the fresh coriander and serve with the brown rice or couscous.

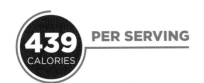 **439 CALORIES PER SERVING**

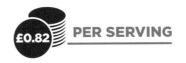 **£0.82 PER SERVING**

SPICED BEAN & LENTIL CHILLI
SERVES 4 ON ITS OWN OR 6 WITH ACCOMPANIMENTS

This is a fun recipe for entertaining – serve it with little bowls of sides (try chopped chillies, roasted sweet potatoes, chopped spring onions and lime wedges). Any leftovers reheat or freeze well. Serve with brown rice or spooned over a baked sweet potato, if your calorie allowance permits.

1 tbsp vegetable oil
1 onion, diced
1 red or orange pepper, diced
3 cloves garlic, finely chopped
2 tsp smoked paprika
2 tsp ground cumin
100g red lentils
1 × 400g tin chopped tomatoes
1 × 400g tin black beans
1 × 400g tin kidney beans
1 avocado, mashed
Juice of ½ lime
85g natural yoghurt
Black pepper

1 Heat the vegetable oil in a heavy-based casserole pan over a medium heat. Add the onion and pepper and sauté for 10 minutes until soft.

2 Turn down the heat slightly, add the garlic and cook for a further 2–3 minutes, stirring regularly to ensure it doesn't burn. Add the paprika and cumin and continue to cook for a further minute, stirring well so the spices coat the vegetables.

3 Add the lentils, tomatoes and 350ml water, bring up to a boil, reduce the heat, cover with a lid and leave to simmer for 15–20 minutes until the lentils are soft.

4 Add the black beans and kidney beans and season with black pepper. If it looks like it's drying out or catching on the bottom of the pan, add a couple of tablespoons more water. Simmer for a further 20 minutes.

5 Meanwhile, mix the mashed avocado with the lime juice in a small bowl and season with black pepper.

6 Serve the chilli in bowls with spoonfuls of the mashed avocado and yoghurt.

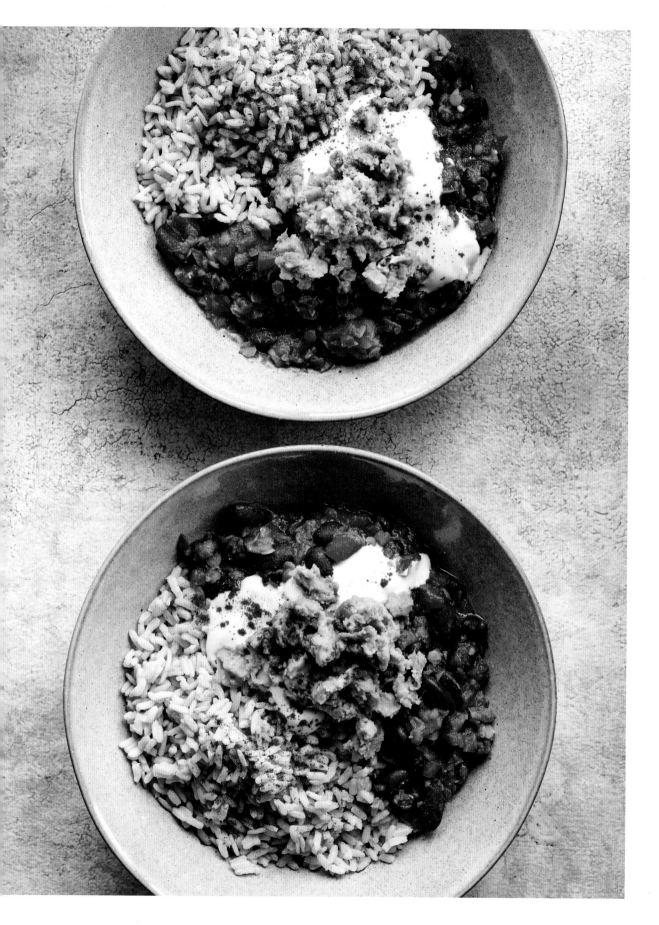

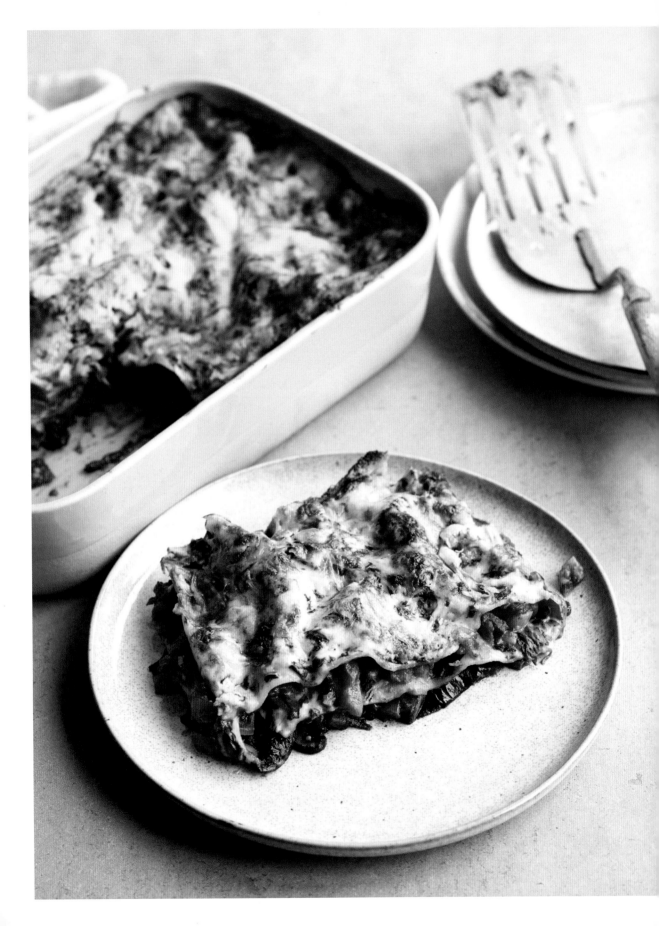

296 CALORIES | PER SERVING

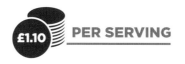

£1.10 | PER SERVING

FIVE VEGETABLE LASAGNE
SERVES 4

A vegetable-packed twist on the classic and a practical dish to have it up your sleeve, as you can prepare this well in advance and simply pop in the oven before serving.

1 small aubergine,
   sliced and chopped
300g mushrooms,
   roughly chopped
3 tbsp vegetable oil
1 onion, finely chopped
3 cloves garlic,
   finely chopped
1 × 400g tin tomatoes
200g roasted peppers from
   a jar, drained and sliced
35g unsalted butter
40g plain flour
300ml semi-skimmed milk
150g spinach
   (fresh or frozen)
20g Cheddar, grated
85g lasagne sheets (or
   enough for two layers)
Black pepper

1 Preheat the oven to 200°C/Fan 180°C.

2 Place the aubergine and mushrooms in a roasting tray and drizzle with 2 tablespoons of the oil, ensuring the vegetables are well coated. Roast in the oven for 45 minutes, until golden brown and soft.

3 Meanwhile, heat the remaining oil in a frying pan over a medium to high heat and add the onion. Sauté for 5 minutes, or until soft. Turn down the heat and add the garlic. Cook for a further 2–3 minutes, stirring regularly to ensure it doesn't burn.

4 Add the tinned tomatoes and roasted peppers, season with black pepper and leave to simmer for 10–15 minutes.

5 Meanwhile, melt the butter in another pan over a medium heat. Add the flour and mix well. Cook for 1–2 minutes then start adding the milk, bit by bit, stirring all the time to avoid lumps.

6 If using fresh spinach, either wilt the spinach in the microwave (place in a bowl and cook on high for 1–2 minutes) or on the hob (place in a covered pan

Recipe continued overleaf

over a medium heat with 2 tablespoons of water for 2–3 minutes). Drain well to remove any excess moisture, then chop the spinach before stirring into the white sauce. If using frozen spinach, either defrost in the microwave (place in a bowl and cook on high for 1–2 minutes) or place in a sieve over the sink and pour boiling water over the top. Drain well to remove any excess moisture, then stir into the sauce.

7 To assemble the lasagne, spoon the roast mushrooms and aubergine into the base of a large ovenproof dish. Pour half the tomato and pepper sauce over the top. Cover with a single layer of lasagne sheets then spread half the spinach sauce over the top. Repeat the layers – tomato and pepper sauce, lasagne sheets and spinach sauce – then top with the grated cheese. Bake in the oven for 35–40 minutes, until golden brown, bubbling and cooked through.

8 Serve with a green salad.

SHOP SAVVY VEGETABLES

Frozen vegetables are convenient and cheap and can be a cost-effective way to mix things up when you can't afford to spend a fortune on fresh fruit and veg. Eating vegetables that are in season can also help to keep the costs down.

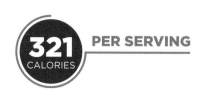
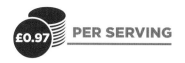
MUSHROOM & BUTTERBEAN BURGERS WITH SWEET POTATO WEDGES

SERVES 4

This is a really hearty, vegetable-based meal. The miso and quinoa give a protein boost and add lots of flavour. The burgers are really delicious with some melted Cheddar on top and served with lots of crisp lettuce and tomato. Make the meal more fun for the younger family members by putting some toppings in little bowls on the table and letting them help themselves. The sweet potato wedges are the perfect accompaniment and would go really well with any grilled meat or fish too.

For the burgers
1 tbsp vegetable oil
6 Portobello or other large
   flat mushrooms (approx.
   500g), roughly chopped
100g cooked quinoa
1 tbsp miso paste
¼ × 400g tin butterbeans,
   drained
75g panko breadcrumbs
Toppings: Cheddar, avocado
   or tomato slices, lettuce
   or gherkins (optional)
Black pepper

For the sweet potato wedges
2 large sweet potatoes,
   cut into thin wedges
1 tbsp cornflour
1 tbsp vegetable oil

1 To make the burgers, heat the vegetable oil in a large frying pan over a medium to high heat. Add the mushrooms and sauté for 15 minutes until soft and brown. Remove from the heat and leave to cool a little.

2 Place the cooled mushrooms, quinoa, miso paste and butterbeans in a food processor and whizz briefly. Tip the mixture into a large bowl, add the panko breadcrumbs and mix through. Season with black pepper then divide the mixture into four and shape into burgers. Place in the fridge to firm up for at least 30 minutes.

3 Preheat the oven to 220°C/Fan 200°C and line a baking tray with baking parchment.

Recipe continued overleaf

4 Place the sweet potato wedges in a large bowl with the cornflour and oil, and mix well with your hands so that each piece of potato is coated.

5 Lay the wedges on an unlined baking tray (making sure you don't overcrowd it) and cook in the oven for 30–35 minutes, turning the wedges halfway through the cooking time.

6 Meanwhile, place the mushroom burgers on the prepared tray and cook for 20 minutes until golden brown, turning halfway through the cooking time. If you like cheese on your burger, top with a slice of cheese 5 minutes before the end of the cooking time.

7 Serve the burgers with a portion of wedges, a green salad and seasoned with plenty of black pepper.

🧺 SHOP SAVVY
PANKO BREADCRUMBS

Once open, you can store panko breadcrumbs in an airtight container and they will keep for up to 6 months. They are great for making breaded fish or chicken goujons – simply cut the raw fish or chicken into bite-sized chunks and then coat in flour, egg and breadcrumbs, as in the recipe for Chicken Schnitzel on page 138.

BEANS

Beans are the ultimate bargain source of protein and fibre and they also release energy slowly. The balance of complex carbohydrates and protein provides a slow, steady source of glucose, instead of the sudden surge that can occur after eating simple carbohydrates. Always go for own brands and spice them up for breakfast, lunch or dinner. If you buy tinned pulses, check the label and choose products that have no added salt or sugar.

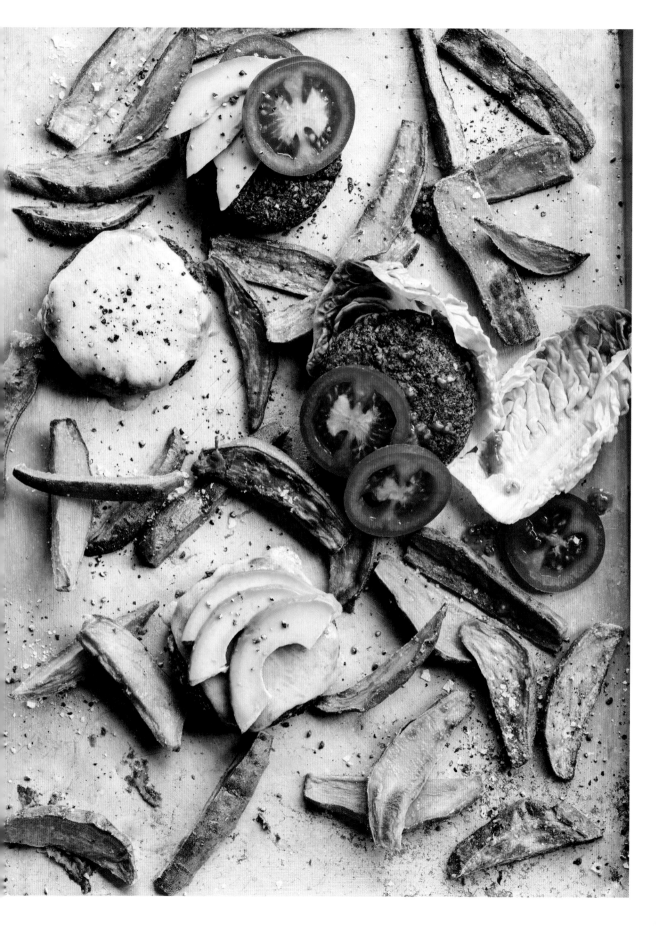

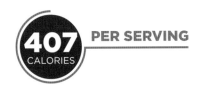

407 CALORIES **PER SERVING**

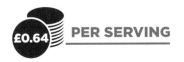

£0.64 **PER SERVING**

LENTIL & TOMATO BOLOGNAISE
SERVES 4

Lentils are a great way to make meat go further. This freezes really well and is delicious served on its own with lots of green veg or with brown rice.

1 tbsp vegetable oil
250g beef mince
1 onion, finely chopped
2 carrots, finely chopped
2 cloves garlic, finely
   chopped
200g brown lentils
1 × 400g tin chopped
   tomatoes
350ml beef stock
   (fresh or made using
   1 low-salt stock cube)
320g wholewheat spaghetti
Black pepper

1 Heat the oil in a large pan over a high heat. Add the beef mince and cook for 5 minutes until brown.

2 Reduce the heat and add the onion and carrot. Sauté gently for 10 minutes, stirring regularly, until the vegetables have started to soften.

3 Stir in the garlic and cook for a further minute.

4 Add the lentils, tinned tomatoes and stock, bring up to a simmer and cook for 30 minutes until the lentils are soft and the flavour has developed.

5 Meanwhile, cook the spaghetti according to the packet instructions. Drain well and set aside.

6 Season the lentils with black pepper and serve with the spaghetti.

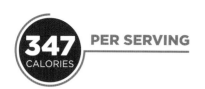
347
CALORIES
PER SERVING

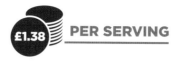
£1.38
PER SERVING

AROMATIC CHICKEN & RICE BROTH
SERVES 4

This is a great recipe to cook when you have a bit of time. The hands-on prep is minimal – it just requires a little bit of chopping then it will simmer away slowly.

1 whole chicken
(approx. 1.4kg)
1 low-salt chicken
stock cube
1 onion, roughly chopped
6cm piece of fresh root
ginger, peeled and
finely sliced
1 cinnamon stick
5 cloves garlic, crushed
Pinch of chilli flakes
175g brown rice
250g mushrooms, sliced
150g green beans, sliced
in half lengthways
2 tbsp miso paste
Black pepper

1 Place the chicken in a large, heavy-based pan that has a lid and pour over 2–3 litres of water (depending on the capacity of your pan), ensuring that the majority of the chicken is covered. Add the stock cube, onion, ginger, cinnamon, garlic and chilli flakes. Place the pan over a high heat and bring to the boil. Reduce the heat, cover with a lid and simmer for 45 minutes, or until the chicken is cooked through.

2 Remove the chicken from the broth and set aside to rest. Meanwhile, turn the heat up under the pan and let the broth bubble away for 15–20 minutes.

3 Cook the rice according to the packet instructions.

4 Shred the chicken meat from the carcass and add approximately 75g chicken to each serving bowl. Save the rest of the meat for further meals, and you could use the chicken carcass to make another stock.

5 Add the mushrooms and green beans to the broth, season with black pepper and simmer for a further 5 minutes before finally adding the cooked rice and miso paste. Stir until everything is combined.

6 Ladle the broth over the chicken in the serving bowls and serve.

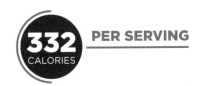
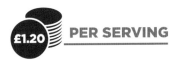
TURKEY MEATBALLS WITH TOMATO SAUCE
SERVES 4

Turkey mince is a great substitute for beef and brings down the calories. Serve these with brown rice, spaghetti or a big green salad, depending on your calorie allowance.

For the meatballs
2 tbsp vegetable oil
1 onion, finely chopped
2 cloves garlic, finely chopped
400g turkey mince
1 egg, beaten
1 tbsp breadcrumbs
Black pepper

For the sauce
1 tbsp vegetable oil
1 bulb of fennel, finely sliced
2 cloves garlic, finely chopped
1 × 400g tin tomatoes
75g sundried tomatoes from
   a jar, roughly chopped
Black pepper

BREADCRUMBS
If you have any stale bread, whizz it in a food processor and store in the freezer for when you need breadcrumbs. No waste and a great way to save money!

1 To make the meatballs, heat 1 tablespoon of the oil in a pan over a medium heat and add the onion. Sauté for 5–10 minutes until soft. Set aside to cool.

2 Combine the cooked onion with the garlic, turkey mince, egg and breadcrumbs in a large bowl and mix well (I find this easiest to do with my hands). Shape the mixture into meatballs and set aside.

3 Heat the remaining oil in a large frying pan over a medium–high heat. Add the meatballs and fry for 2 minutes, turning them to colour each side. Don't worry about cooking them through. Once golden, remove the pan from the heat and set aside.

4 To make the sauce, heat the oil in a saucepan over a medium heat and sauté the fennel for 10 minutes until soft. Add the garlic and cook for 2–3 minutes, stirring regularly to ensure it doesn't burn. Stir in the tinned and sundried tomatoes and 100ml water, season with black pepper and simmer for 15–20 minutes, adding more water if it starts to dry out.

5 Pour the sauce into the frying pan with the meatballs and place over a medium heat. Simmer gently for 5–10 minutes, until the meatballs are cooked through.

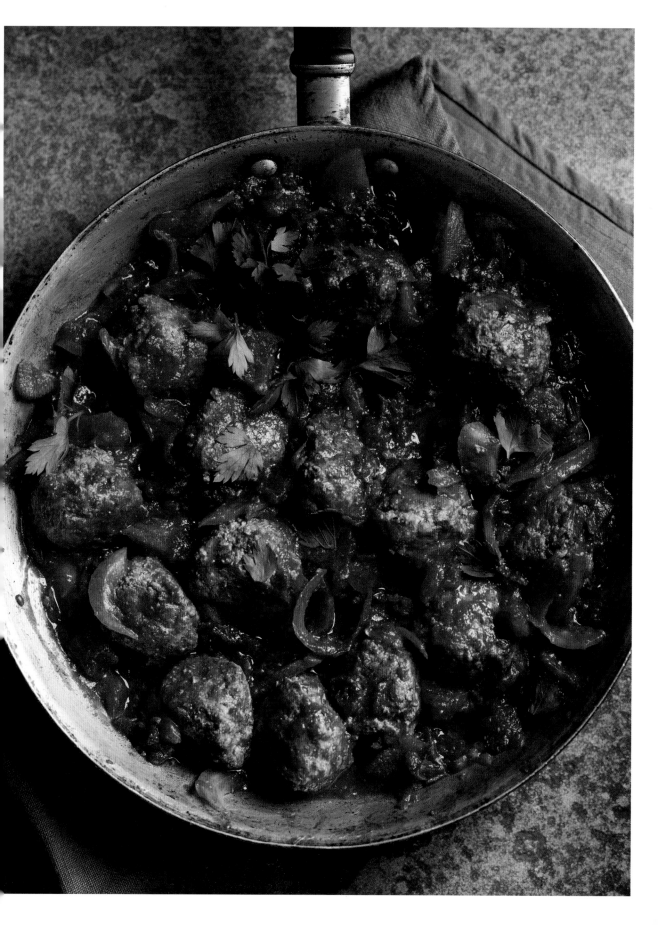

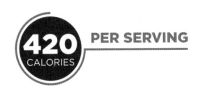
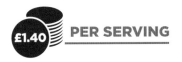

CHICKEN SCHNITZEL WITH THREE VEG SLAW
SERVES 4

These schnitzels are a hit with the whole family and are a great dish to prepare ahead. Store them in the fridge or freezer (individually wrapped) and simply defrost and fry them when you're ready.

For the schnitzel
4 skinless and boneless
    chicken breasts
50g plain flour
1 egg, beaten
1 tbsp semi-skimmed milk
100g panko breadcrumbs
20g Parmesan, grated
1 tbsp vegetable oil
Black pepper

For the slaw
50g kale, sliced
1 tbsp olive oil
Juice of 1 lemon
2 carrots, peeled into
    ribbons
½ small red cabbage
    (approx. 250g),
    finely sliced
125g natural yoghurt
1 tsp Dijon mustard
1 small clove garlic,
    finely chopped
Black pepper

1 To make the slaw, place the kale in a large bowl, add the olive oil and lemon juice and season with black pepper. Massage with your fingertips until the kale has started to wilt. Add the carrot, cabbage, yoghurt, mustard and garlic and mix well. Cover and set aside.

2 Place clingfilm on the work surface and lay the chicken breasts on top. Place another piece of clingfilm over the top and, using a rolling pin, bash the chicken to flatten until roughly 2–3mm thick.

3 Measure the flour on to a plate and season with black pepper. Place the egg and milk in a shallow bowl and mix with a fork. Mix the breadcrumbs with the Parmesan on another plate. Dip each chicken breast in the seasoned flour, turning it over to ensure it is fully covered. Next, dip into the egg and milk mixture then, finally, dip into the breadcrumbs until completely covered. At this stage you can cover them and refrigerate until needed.

4 Heat the vegetable oil in a large, non-stick frying pan over a medium–high heat. Cook the schnitzels for 2–3 minutes on each side until golden brown and cooked through. Serve with the slaw.

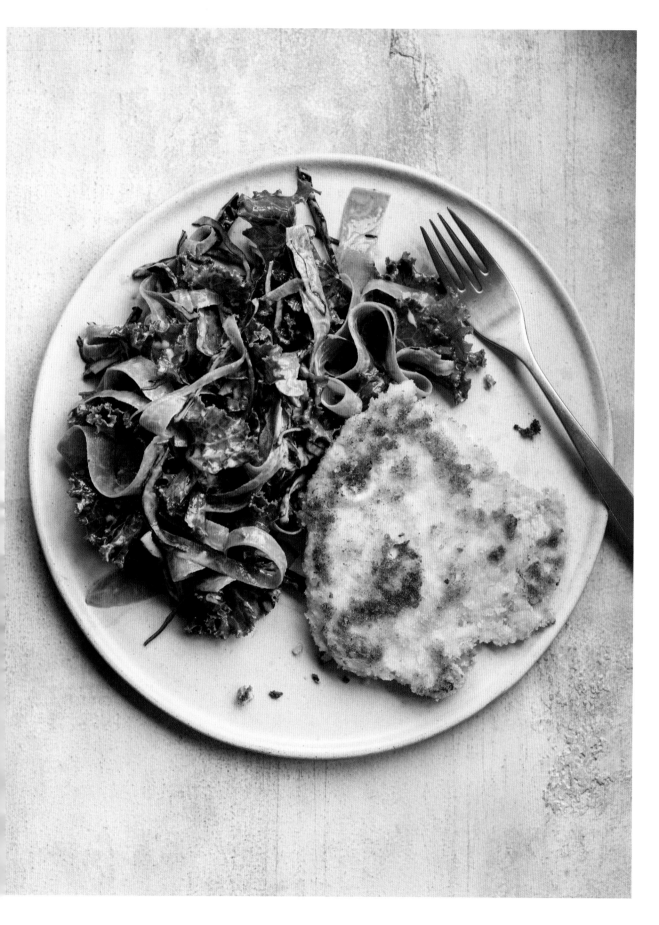

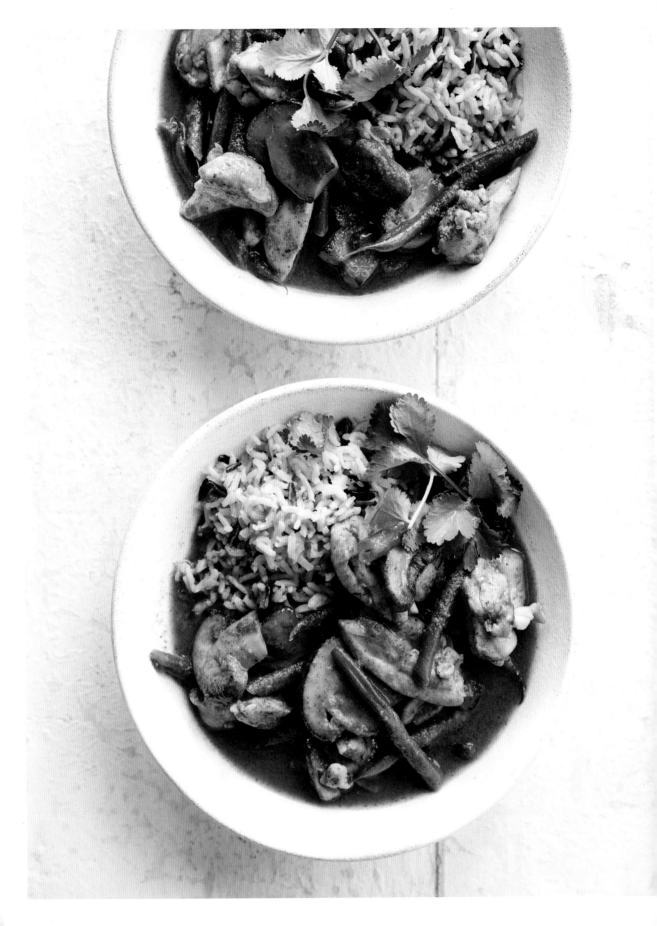

439 CALORIES **PER SERVING**

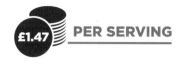

£1.47 **PER SERVING**

EASY THAI GREEN CURRY
SERVES 4

Instead of splurging on a takeaway, make this fresh and zingy curry. If you're making it for kids leave out the chilli. You could swap the chicken for any firm white fish or prawns. You could even make it vegetarian by using extra veg and adding a tin of chickpeas or butterbeans.

300g brown rice
1 tbsp vegetable oil
1 onion, roughly chopped
3 cloves garlic, peeled
2.5cm piece of fresh
    root ginger, peeled
Zest and juice of 1 lime
30g fresh coriander
½–1 chilli (to taste)
4 skinless, boneless
    chicken thighs, chopped
    into bite-sized pieces
200g chestnut mushrooms,
    sliced
1 × 400ml tin coconut milk
4 tsp cornflour
200g green beans
Black pepper

1 Cook the rice according to the packet instructions.

2 Meanwhile, place the vegetable oil, onion, garlic, ginger, lime zest and juice, coriander and chilli in a food processor with some black pepper and whizz until smooth.

3 Place a heavy-based saucepan over a medium heat, add the paste and cook for 3–4 minutes, stirring so it doesn't burn or stick. Add the chicken pieces and mushrooms and continue to cook for 3–4 minutes, until golden. Pour in the coconut milk and 200ml water. Combine the cornflour with 2 tablespoons of water in a small bowl, then pour this into the pan, stirring well. Bring to a gentle simmer, reduce the heat and cook for 10 minutes, until the chicken is cooked through and the sauce has thickened.

4 Finally, add the green beans and cook for a final 2–3 minutes.

5 Serve in bowls with the brown rice.

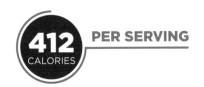
412 CALORIES **PER SERVING**

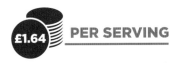
£1.64 **PER SERVING**

SPANISH CHICKEN & CHORIZO STEW
SERVES 4

This hearty Mediterranean stew is a great winter warmer. It's quick and easy to make and is cooked all in one pot so there is minimal washing up.

1 tbsp vegetable oil
1 red onion, finely sliced
150g chorizo sausage, sliced
4 skinless and boneless
  chicken thighs,
  roughly chopped
1 red pepper, sliced
2 tsp smoked paprika
4 cloves garlic, finely
  chopped
1 × 400g tin chopped
  tomatoes
250ml chicken stock
  (fresh or made using
  1 low-salt stock cube)
1 × 400g tin chickpeas,
  drained
15g fresh flat-leaf parsley,
  chopped
Black pepper

1 Heat the oil in a casserole dish over a medium heat. Add the onion and sauté for 5 minutes or until soft.

2 Turn up the heat, add the chorizo to the pan and cook for 2–3 minutes, stirring regularly to ensure it doesn't burn.

3 Reduce the heat, add the chicken, pepper, paprika and garlic and cook for another 2–3 minutes.

4 Pour in the tinned tomatoes and chicken stock, season with black pepper and leave to simmer for 15 minutes.

5 Add the chickpeas to the pan and simmer for another 5 minutes.

6 Remove from the heat, stir through the parsley and serve with steamed veg.

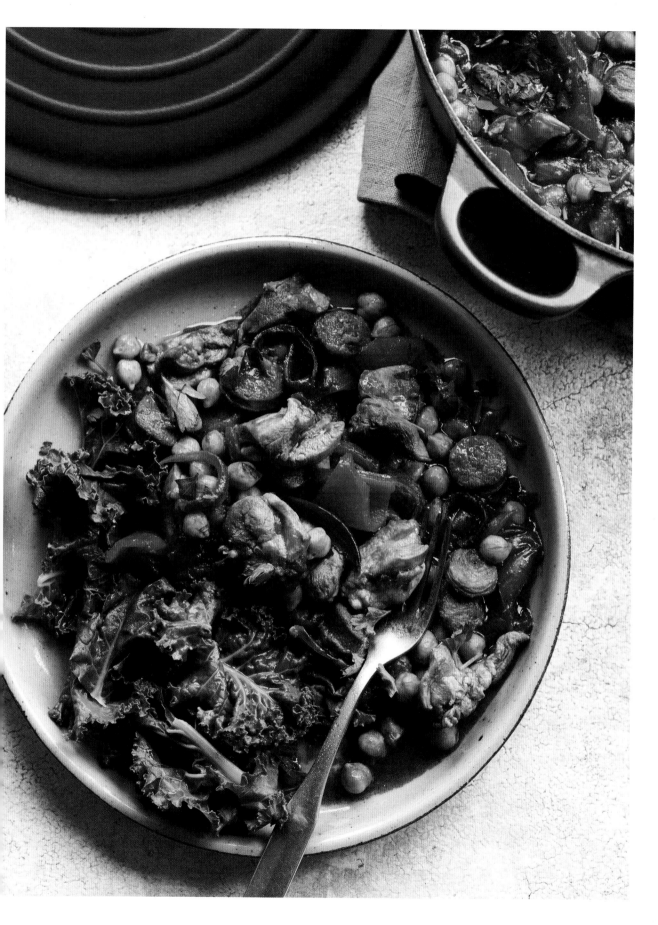

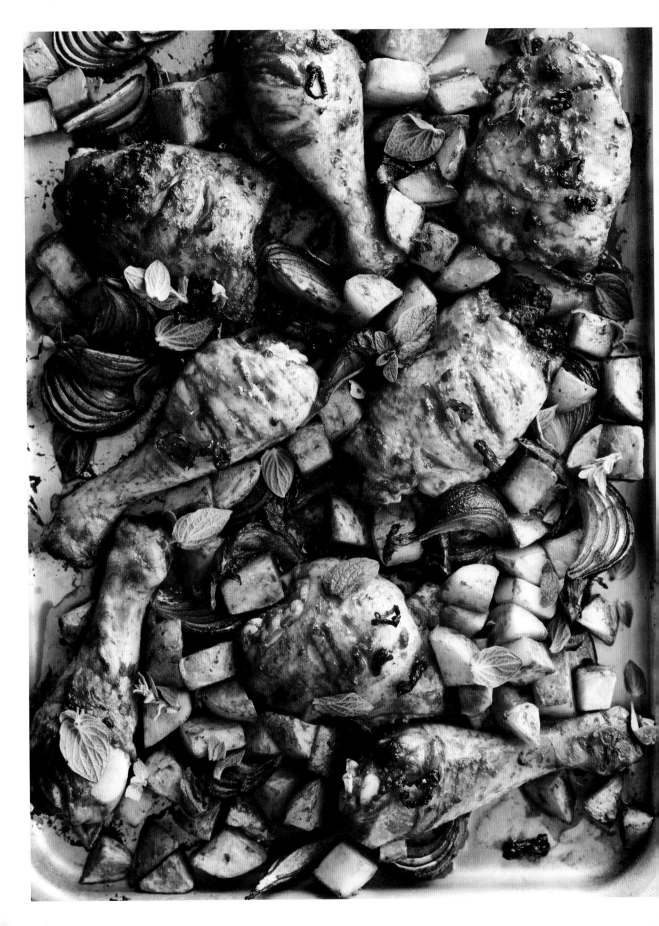

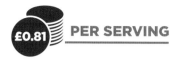
PERI PERI CHICKEN WITH CRISPY POTATOES
SERVES 4

This traditional fiery chicken recipe has had a low-cal and mild make-over. Great for all the family, you can remove the chilli if you're cooking for kids.

3 tbsp vegetable oil
4 tsp smoked paprika
4 cloves garlic, finely
  chopped
4 tbsp tomato purée
2 tsp dried oregano or
  1 tbsp fresh oregano
2 tsp brown sugar or honey
1 red chilli, finely sliced
4 chicken thighs
4 chicken drumsticks
2 red onions, cut
  into wedges
800g potatoes, peeled
  and chopped
  into bite-sized pieces
Fresh flat-leaf parsley or
  oregano, to serve
  (optional)
Black pepper

1 Preheat the oven to 200°C/Fan 180°C.

2 Make the marinade by combining 2 tablespoons of the vegetable oil with the smoked paprika, garlic, tomato purée, oregano, brown sugar, chilli and some black pepper in a small mixing bowl.

3 Place the chicken thighs, drumsticks and red onions in a large dish. Pour the marinade over the top and mix well to make sure the chicken and onions are well coated. Leave to marinate for at least 1 hour, preferably longer (ideally overnight in the fridge).

4 Place the chopped potatoes on a baking tray and drizzle with the remaining 1 tablespoon of vegetable oil. Season with black pepper and toss to ensure the potatoes are well coated in the oil. Place in the oven. After 5 minutes, remove the potatoes from the oven and add the chicken and onions to the tray. Return to the oven and cook for 30–35 minutes until the chicken is cooked through and the potatoes are golden and crispy.

5 Serve with a crunchy green salad.

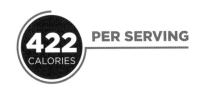
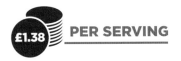
SALMON WITH CREAMY POTATO, CUCUMBER, DILL & RADISH SALAD

SERVES 4

A fresh and nutritious recipe, the cucumber, dill and radishes go really well together. This would also be delicious eaten cold, making it ideal for a packed lunch, too.

500g new potatoes,
   halved
4 salmon fillets
   (approx. 120g)
Zest and juice of 1 lemon
½ cucumber, diced
150g radishes, finely sliced
15g fresh dill,
   roughly chopped
2 tbsp natural yoghurt
1 tbsp olive oil
Black pepper

1 Preheat the oven to 200°C/Fan 180°C and line a baking tray with foil.

2 Cook the potatoes in boiling water for 20 minutes or until tender. Drain and set aside in a large bowl to cool for 10–15 minutes.

3 Place the salmon fillets on the prepared baking tray and season with black pepper. Pour the lemon juice over the salmon and bake in the oven for 20 minutes.

4 Meanwhile, add the cucumber, radishes, dill, yoghurt, lemon zest and olive oil to the bowl with the potatoes. Season with black pepper and mix to combine.

5 Serve the salmon fillets with the potato, dill and radish salad on the side with some steamed greens.

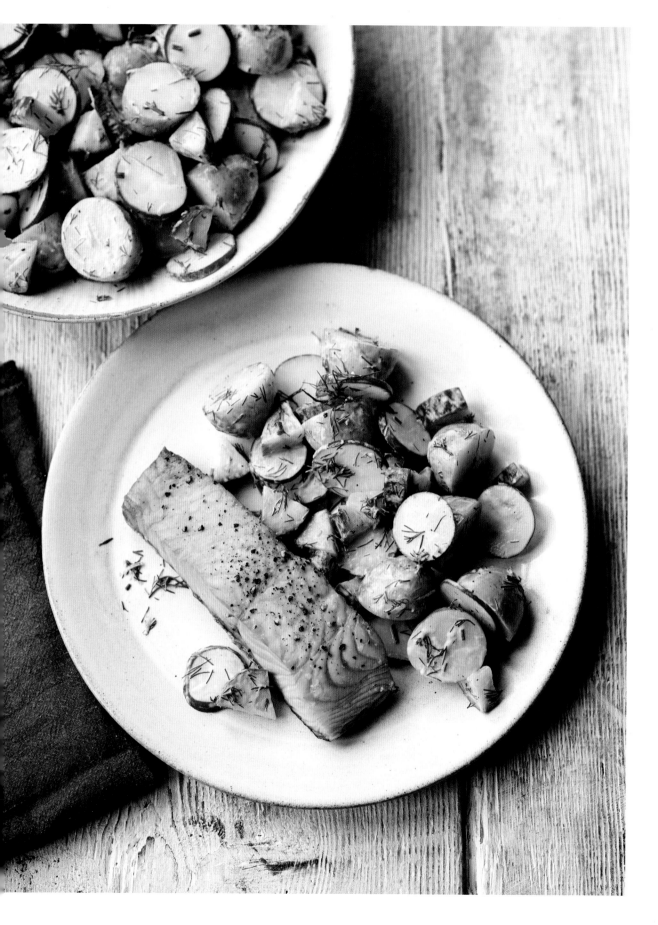

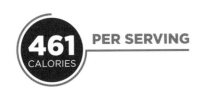
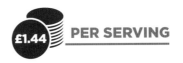

ASIAN SALMON BURGERS WITH PETITS POIS & POTATO MASH

SERVES 4

This is a great way to serve salmon and also a clever way to introduce the fish to kids who may be a little fussy.

4 salmon fillets (approx. 120g), skin removed
1 tsp low-salt soy sauce
15g fresh coriander, roughly chopped
1 tbsp sesame oil
Zest of 1 lime
1 bunch of spring onions, sliced
700g potatoes, peeled and roughly chopped
150g petits pois
1 tbsp vegetable oil
2 tbsp semi-skimmed milk
Lime wedges, to serve
Black pepper

1 Place the salmon fillets in a food processor with the soy sauce, coriander, sesame oil, lime zest, spring onions, reserving a handful to garnish, and some black pepper. Pulse 4–5 times until you have a coarse mince – do not over blitz at this stage or it will be difficult to form into burgers. Rub a little oil on to the palms of your hands to prevent sticking and shape the salmon mixture into 4 burgers. Refrigerate for at least 30 minutes to firm.

2 Meanwhile, place the potatoes in a pan of water over a high heat. Bring to the boil, reduce the heat and simmer for 10 minutes. Add the peas and cook for a further 5 minutes. Drain and return the potato and pea mixture to the pan, adding a drizzle of oil, the milk and some black pepper. Mash well and set aside.

3 Just before cooking the burgers, drizzle a little vegetable oil over them, using your heads to rub it over evenly. Place a frying pan over a medium–high heat and cook the burgers for approximately 5–6 minutes on each side, until they are firm to the touch, brown and cooked through.

4 Sprinkle with the reserved spring onion and serve with the mash and lime wedges.

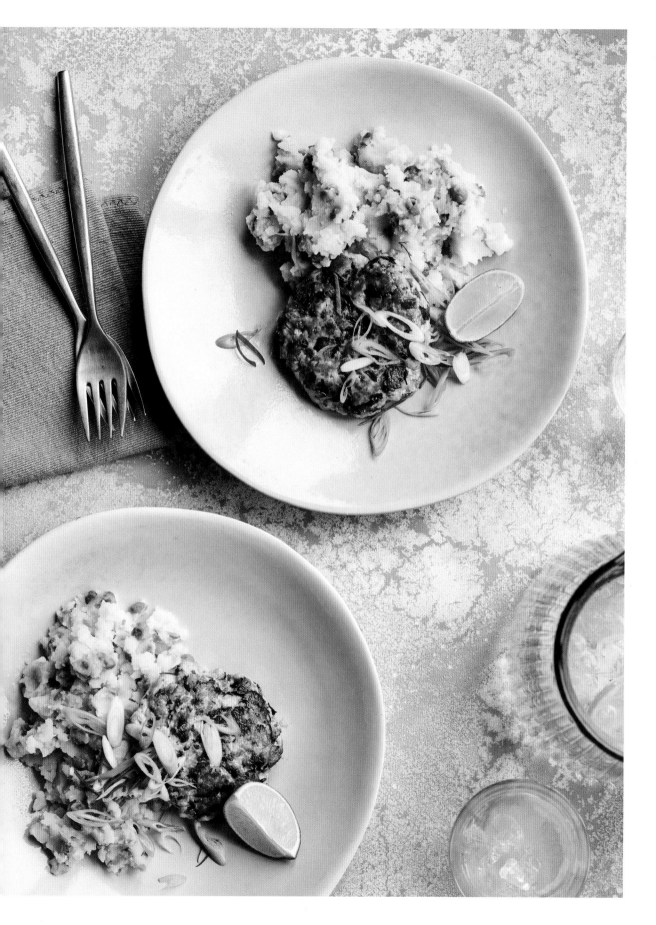

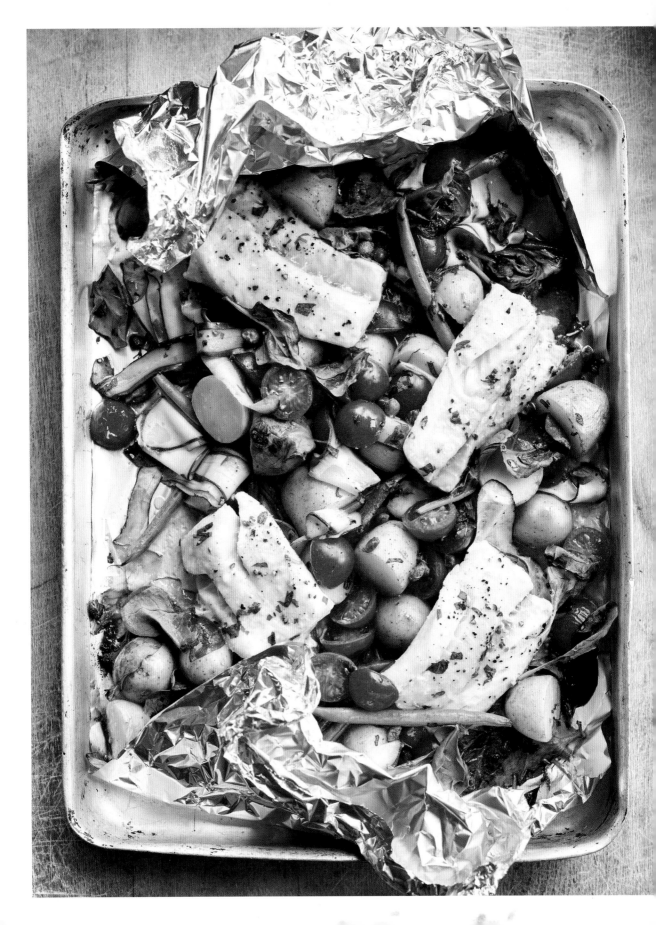

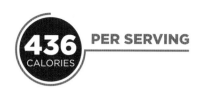 **PER SERVING**

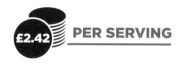 **PER SERVING**

SUPER EASY FISH TRAY BAKE
SERVES 4

This is an ideal midweek dinner when you are time poor but want something healthy and filling. You can use frozen fish here – it is really cost effective to buy bags of frozen fish fillets and keep them in the freezer, as opposed to buying fresh fish all the time. Just make sure you up the cooking time to 25 minutes if you are cooking the fish from frozen.

700g new potatoes, halved if big
200g green beans
30g fresh basil, finely chopped
50g capers, drained and finely chopped
Juice of 1 lemon
3 tbsp olive oil
2 courgettes, grated or peeled into ribbons
300g cherry tomatoes, halved
150g fresh spinach
4 cod fillets (approx. 120g) (any firm white fish will work here)
Black pepper

1 Preheat the oven to 220°C/Fan 200°C and line a large baking tray with a layer of foil, with enough overhang to wrap it up into a parcel.

2 Bring a large pan of water to the boil and cook the potatoes for 10 minutes. Add the green beans to the pan for the final 4 minutes of the cooking time. Drain and set aside.

3 In a large bowl, combine the basil, capers, lemon juice and 2 tablespoons of the olive oil. Add the courgettes, cherry tomatoes, spinach, cooked potatoes and beans. Mix everything together well and season with black pepper.

4 Tip the vegetable mixture on to the tray and spread out evenly, leaving enough space at the edges to fold the foil over and close. Lay the cod fillets on top of the vegetables and drizzle with the remaining olive oil. Season with black pepper, bring the edges of the foil together to seal into a parcel and bake in the oven for 15–25 minutes (depending on whether the fish is fresh or frozen).

5 Divide the vegetables between four plates and top with a cod fillet to serve.

PER SERVING

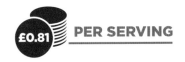
PER SERVING

PEARL BARLEY, BACON & KALE WARMER
SERVES 4

A quick and easy, warming stew that is great for dinner on a cold winter night. Pearl barley is a thrifty ingredient, good to have in the store cupboard to bulk out soups and stews.

1 tbsp vegetable oil
1 onion, diced
3 carrots, diced
8 rashers unsmoked back
 bacon, thinly sliced
2 cloves garlic,
 finely chopped
15g fresh thyme, leaves
 picked and finely chopped
300g pearl barley
1l chicken stock (fresh or
 made with 2 low-salt
 stock cubes)
250g kale, chopped
Parmesan, grated, to serve
Black pepper

1 Heat the oil in a large pan over a medium heat. Add the onion and carrots and cook for 10 minutes until soft. Turn the heat up and add the bacon. Fry for a further 5 minutes until it is starting to brown, stirring regularly to ensure it doesn't burn.

2 Turn the heat down, add the garlic and thyme leaves and cook for 2 minutes. Stir in the pearl barley and pour in the stock. Cover with a lid and simmer for 45 minutes or until the pearl barley is tender.

3 Finally, stir in the kale and cook for a further 5 minutes until the kale is tender. Season with black pepper and serve with a little Parmesan grated over the top.

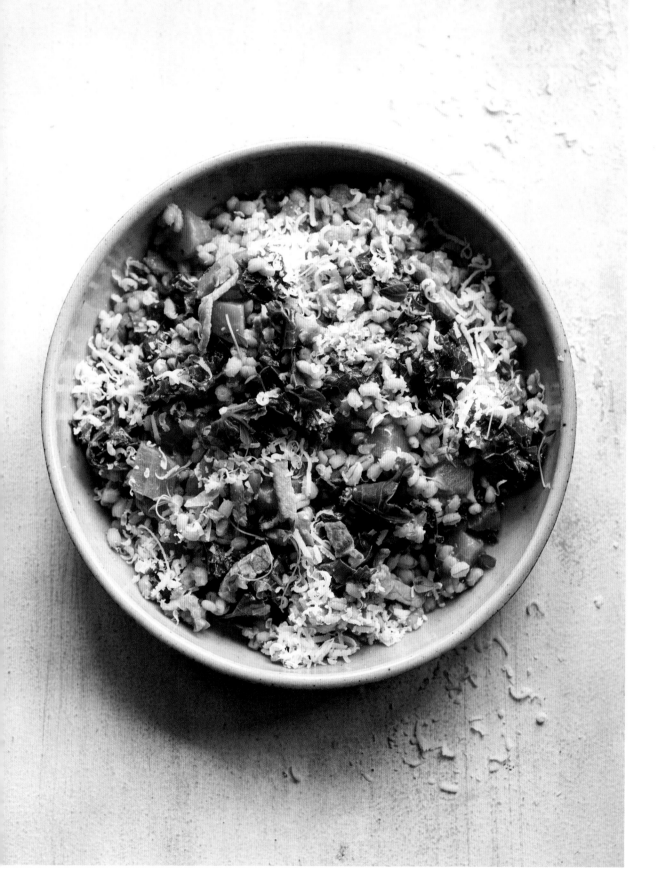

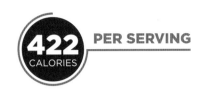
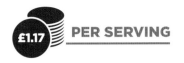
CHINESE PORK NOODLES
SERVES 4

Minced pork is a good low-fat and low-cost option, and is perfect in a stir-fry. This is a delicious and speedy midweek meal that the whole family will enjoy.

1 tbsp vegetable oil
500g lean pork mince
2 tsp Chinese 5 spice
2 cloves garlic,
    finely chopped
200g mushrooms, sliced
6 spring onions, finely sliced
2 tbsp low-salt soy sauce
1 tbsp honey
150g sugar snap peas
150g egg noodles
Juice of 1 lime
Black pepper

1 Heat the oil in a wok or large frying pan over a high heat. Add the pork mince and fry until browned.

2 Reduce the heat then add the Chinese 5 spice, garlic, mushrooms and spring onions and fry for 5 minutes.

3 Stir in the soy sauce, honey, sugar snap peas and a splash of water and cook for a further 5 minutes, stirring occasionally, until the sugar snap peas are cooked.

4 Meanwhile, cook the noodles according to the packet instructions. Drain well and set aside.

5 Finally, mix the noodles into the pork and veg mixture, stir in the lime juice, season with black pepper and serve.

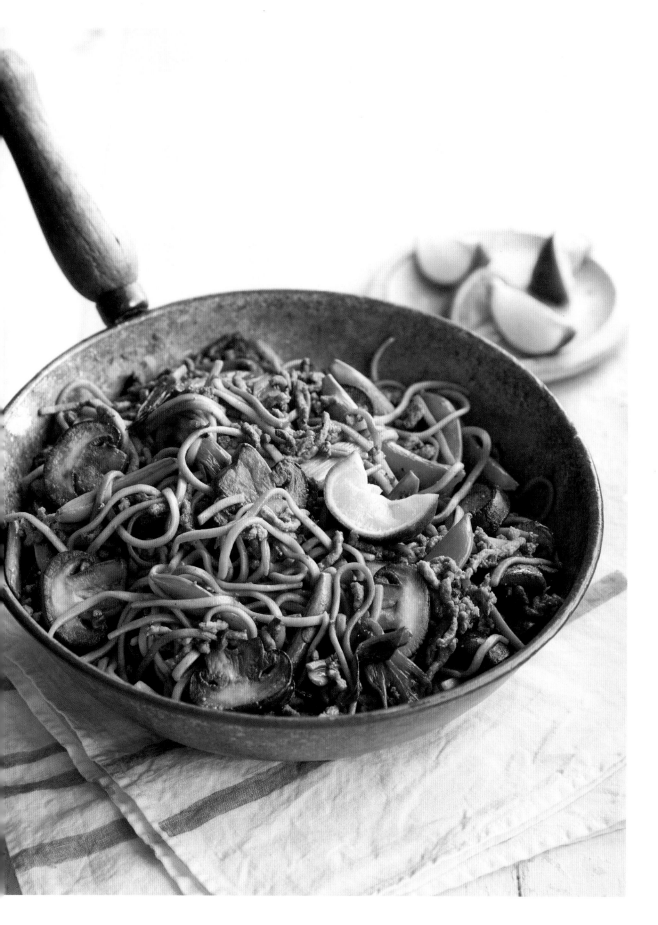

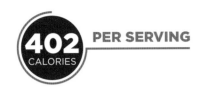 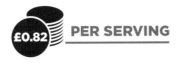

ZINGY COURGETTE CARBONARA
SERVES 4

Pasta is such a crowd pleaser! In this recipe, some of the pasta has been replaced with thinly sliced courgettes and it still tastes delicious. You can also use the biggest setting on a grater to make the courgette ribbons.

200g wholewheat spaghetti
1 tbsp olive oil
6 rashers unsmoked streaky bacon, roughly chopped
3 cloves garlic, finely chopped
2 eggs, beaten
Zest and juice of ½ lemon
60g Parmesan, grated
3 large courgettes (approx. 500g), thinly sliced lengthways/ spiralised, peeled with a julienne peeler
Black pepper

1 Cook the spaghetti according to the packet instructions. Drain well, reserving the cooking water, and set aside.

2 Meanwhile, heat the oil in a large frying pan over a medium heat. Add the bacon and fry for 10 minutes until crispy.

3 Turn the heat down, add the garlic and cook for a further minute until fragrant, stirring regularly to ensure it doesn't burn.

4 Meanwhile, in a small bowl, combine the eggs, lemon zest and juice, some black pepper and most of the Parmesan, keeping some back to garnish later.

5 Add the spaghetti and courgettes to the pan with the bacon, mix everything together well, adding a splash more pasta water if it seems at all sticky.

6 When everything is hot through, turn the heat right down and pour in the Parmesan and egg mixture. Stir everything together well, working quickly so you don't scramble the eggs.

7 Divide the pasta between four bowls or plates and sprinkle with the reserved Parmesan and some black pepper to serve.

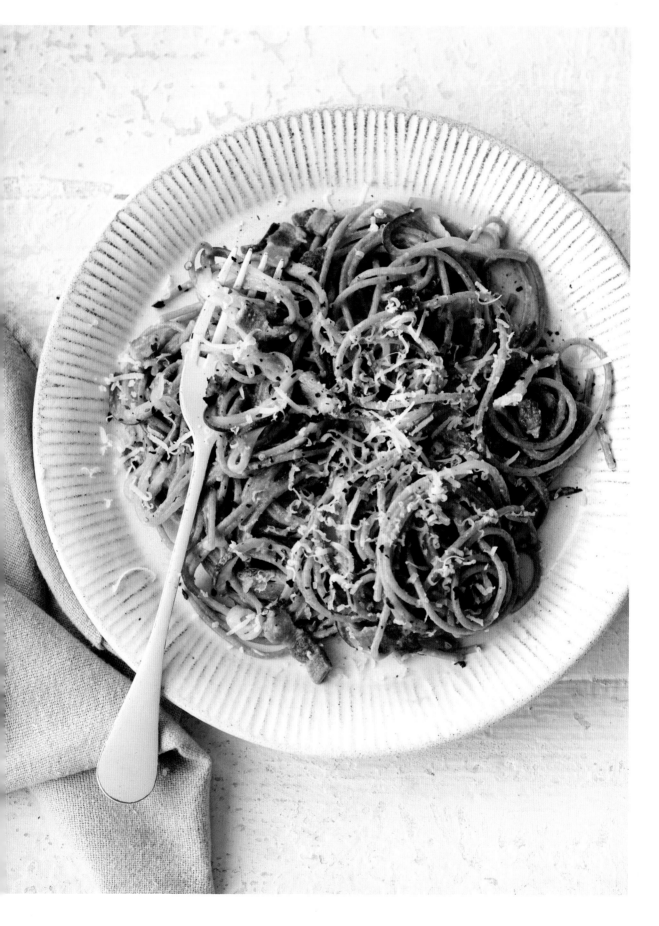

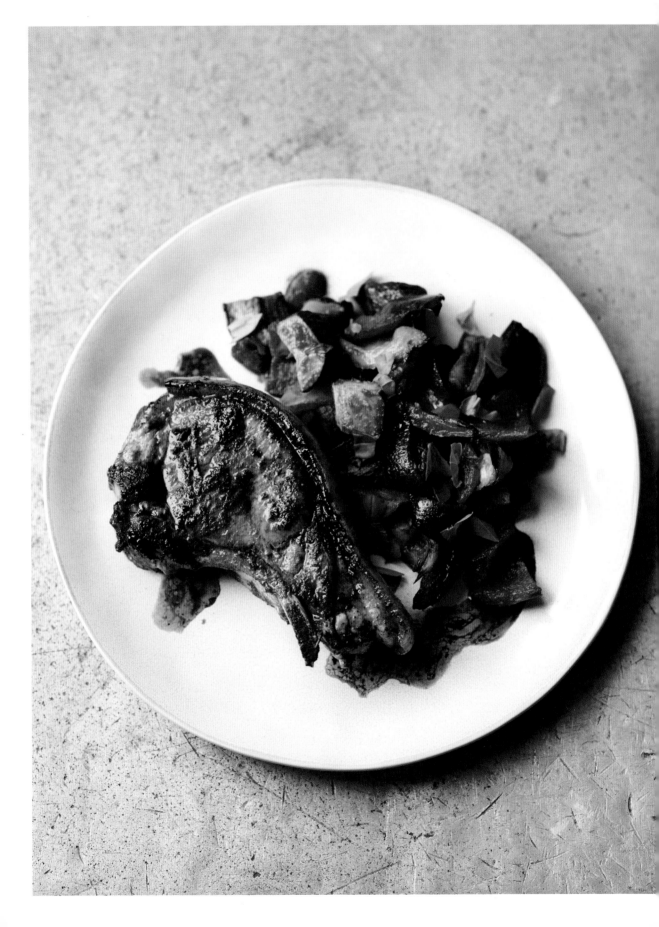

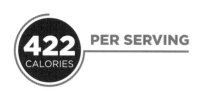
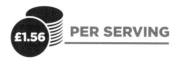
PORK CHOPS WITH ROAST VEGETABLE RATATOUILLE

SERVES 4

The roast vegetable ratatouille is a great way to help you reach your 5 a day. It's a perfect side dish for any grilled meat or fish. The paprika rub on the pork chops gives a delicious crust as it grills.

2 courgettes, roughly chopped
2 red or orange peppers, roughly chopped
1 aubergine, roughly chopped
1 red onion, roughly chopped
3 tbsp vegetable oil
3 cloves garlic, finely chopped
1 × 400g tin chopped tomatoes
2 tsp smoked paprika
4 bone-in pork chops
15g fresh basil, chopped
Black pepper

1 Preheat the oven to 200°C/Fan 180°C.

2 Place the courgettes, peppers, aubergine and red onion in a roasting tin. Drizzle with 1 tablespoon of the oil and season with black pepper. Place in the oven and roast for 30 minutes.

3 Remove the tin from the oven, add the garlic and tinned tomatoes and return to the oven for a further 15 minutes.

4 Meanwhile, mix the remaining vegetable oil with the paprika. Rub the paprika and oil paste into both sides of the pork chops and season with black pepper.

5 Heat a large, non-stick frying pan over a high heat. Add the pork chops and fry for approximately 7 minutes on each side, or until cooked through. Make sure to brown the fat. Remove the pork chops from the pan and leave to rest for a few minutes.

6 Remove the vegetables from the oven and scatter the basil over the top.

7 Serve the pork chops with the roasted vegetables and some steamed greens.

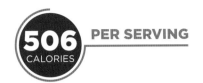 **PER SERVING**

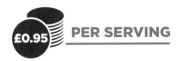 **PER SERVING**

SAUSAGE RAGU WITH BROWN RICE
SERVES 4

The flavours of the sausage and fennel go so well together in this ragu. It's a great way to use up sausages or sausage meat and you could substitute the pork for chicken sausages, if you prefer, to bring down the calorie count. The ragu freezes really well.

1 tbsp vegetable oil
1 red onion, diced
2 celery sticks, diced
2 carrots, diced
8 pork or chicken sausages, skins removed
3 cloves garlic, finely chopped
1 tsp fennel seeds
1 × 400g tin chopped tomatoes
250g brown rice
Black pepper

1 Heat the oil in a large pan over a medium heat. Add the onion, celery and carrot and sauté for 5 minutes. Stir in the sausage meat and turn up the heat. Brown the meat, stirring occasionally.

2 Reduce the heat, add the garlic and fennel seeds and cook for another minute. Stir in the tomatoes, 200ml water and season with black pepper. Bring to the boil then reduce the heat and simmer for 30–40 minutes.

3 Meanwhile, cook the rice according to the packet instructions.

4 Serve the sausage ragu with the rice and a green salad.

 DIET HACK
Do I need to say 'Bye, bye' to salad dressing?

Dressings are still on the menu – as long as you're not overgenerous. A little vinaigrette made with unsaturated oil, such as olive, rapeseed or sunflower, can bring out the flavour of the salad and help to combine the ingredients. You can also add water to make them go further, instead of more oil – just put everything in a jar and shake to mix well. Use garlic, mustard, finely chopped onions, chives or chilli to complement different combinations as well, and this will help to keep the amount of oil you need to use right down.

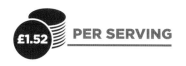

415 CALORIES PER SERVING

£1.52 PER SERVING

SHEPHERD'S PIE WITH VEG MASH TOPPING
SERVES 4

A great twist on the classic that ups your veg intake and lowers the calories. A wonderful prepare-ahead recipe that also reheats and freezes really well.

1 tbsp vegetable oil
1 onion, diced
3 celery sticks, diced
500g lean lamb mince
1 × 400g tin chopped tomatoes
300ml stock (fresh or made with 1 low-salt chicken or vegetable stock cube)
1 swede (approx. 450g), peeled and chopped
5 large carrots (approx. 400g), chopped
25g Parmesan, grated
Black pepper

1 Heat the oil in a large non-stick pan over a medium heat. Add the onion and celery and sauté for 10 minutes until soft. Turn up the heat, add the mince and cook for a further 10 minutes until starting to brown, breaking it up with a wooden spoon as it cooks.

2 Add the tomatoes and stock and season with black pepper. Bring to the boil, reduce the heat and leave it to simmer for 35 minutes.

3 Meanwhile, bring a large pan of water to the boil and cook the swede and carrots for 20–25 minutes, or until soft. Drain and leave to cool a little before whizzing in a food processor until you have a smooth purée. Season with black pepper to taste.

4 Preheat the oven to 200°C/Fan 180°C.

5 Spoon the lamb into a medium-sized oven dish, spread the carrot and swede mixture over the top and sprinkle with the Parmesan. Bake in the oven for 30 minutes until piping hot and golden.

6 Serve with steamed greens.

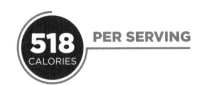 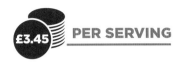

SLOW-COOKED LAMB WITH BUTTERBEAN MASH
SERVES 4 WITH LEFTOVER MEAT

This is so easy to prepare; the oven does all the hard work and the results are melt-in-the mouth delicious. It's a little more expensive and calorific than other roasts but it is good for a treat and better than splurging on a takeaway. You'll have leftover lamb for another meal, too – it is great used as a filling for the Spinach Wraps on page 88).

For the lamb
2kg shoulder of lamb
1 whole head garlic,
  cloves separated
  (no need to peel them)
1 tbsp olive oil
6 sprigs rosemary
400ml stock (fresh or made
  with 1 low-salt chicken
  or vegetable stock cube)
Black pepper

For the butterbean mash
1 tbsp vegetable oil
1 onion, diced
2 cloves garlic,
  finely chopped
2 tsp smoked paprika
2 × 400g tins butterbeans,
  drained
Juice of ½ lemon

1 Preheat the oven to 200°C/Fan 180°C.

2 Place the lamb in a large roasting tin. Make small cuts all over the meat with a knife; this will help infuse the rosemary and garlic flavours. Roughly crush the garlic in a pestle and mortar with the olive oil and some black pepper. Spoon this all over the lamb and lay the rosemary sprigs on top. Pour the stock into the base of the tin, cover everything with foil and roast in the oven for 30 minutes.

3 Turn the oven down to 170°C/Fan 150°C and roast for a further 5 hours. Baste the meat with the juices twice during the cooking time.

4 Meanwhile, to make the mash, heat the oil in a pan over a medium heat. Add the onion and sauté for 10 minutes until soft. Add the garlic and paprika and cook for another 2 minutes, stirring regularly to ensure it doesn't burn. Add the butterbeans, lemon juice and 200ml water and bring to a simmer. Pour into a food processor and whizz until creamy.

5 Remove the lamb from the oven; it should pull apart easily with two forks. Serve 85g lamb per person with the butterbean mash and some steamed greens.

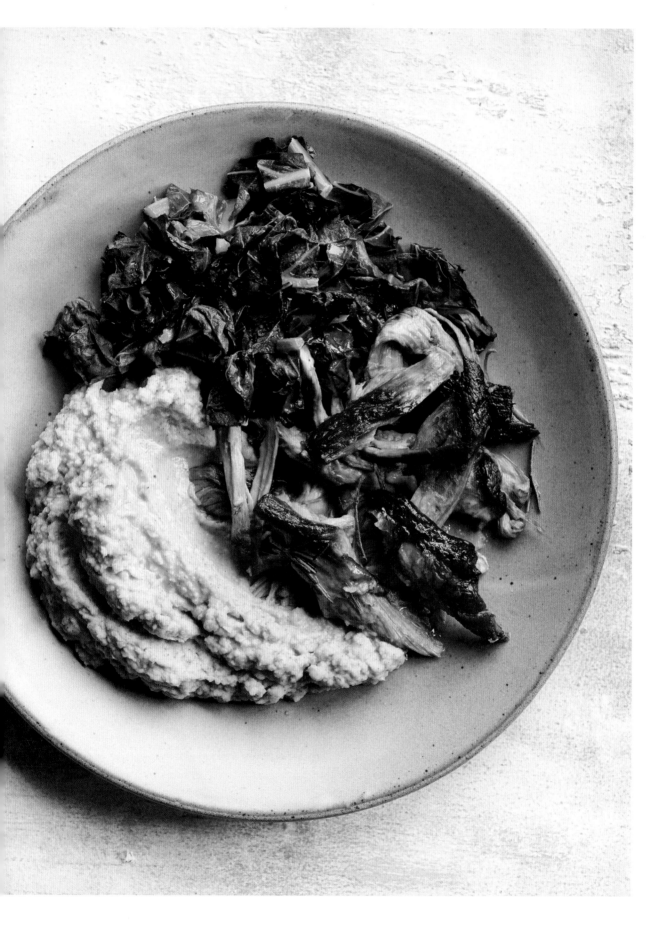

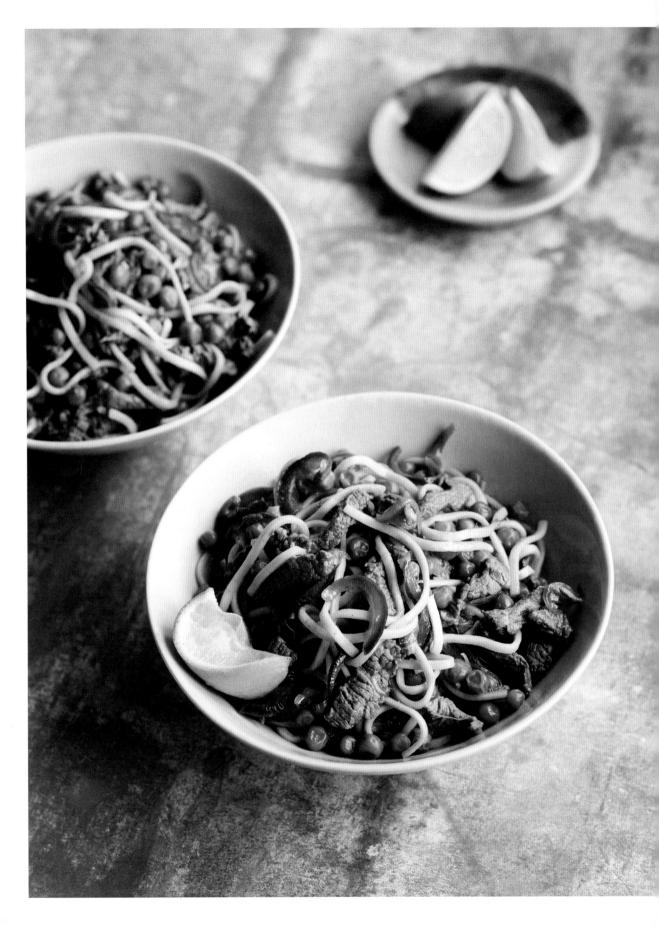

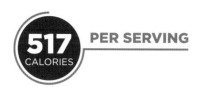

517 CALORIES PER SERVING

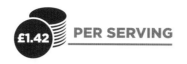

£1.42 PER SERVING

TERIYAKI BEEF & PEA STIR-FRY
SERVES 4

This stir-fry is a great way of making meat go further. It's an easy, speedy dinner that is perfect for the whole family.

1 tbsp vegetable oil
1 red onion, sliced
4 cloves garlic, finely
   chopped
4cm piece of fresh root
   ginger, peeled and
   finely chopped
2 × 150g rump steaks,
   fat removed, cut into
   thin strips
3 tbsp low-salt soy sauce
2 tbsp honey
400g petits pois or frozen
   garden peas
300g egg noodles
1 lime, cut into wedges

1 Heat the oil in a large non-stick frying pan over a medium to high heat. Add the onion, garlic and ginger and cook for 2–3 minutes, stirring regularly.

2 Add the strips of steak and stir-fry for a further 2 minutes. Add the soy sauce, honey, peas and 200ml water and let it bubble away and reduce for a further 2–3 minutes until the peas have cooked.

3 Meanwhile, cook the noodles according to the packet instructions. Drain well and add them to the pan. Mix everything together well then serve immediately with lime wedges.

IS ALL MEAT BAD FOR YOU?
On average, people in the UK eat 70g of red and processed meat (cooked weight) a day. The Department of Health recommends you don't eat more than 90g a day. The amount of saturated fat in different types of meat will vary but processed meats, like bacon, sausages and ham, can come with lots of salt, too. Make sure you read food labels to make a healthier choice. Choose lean cuts of red meat or extra-lean mince to keep the saturated fat content down. Lean cuts of meat may seem more expensive but you can use less. Use lower fat cooking methods like grilling instead of frying, too.

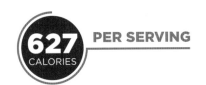 **PER SERVING**

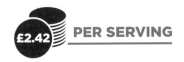 **PER SERVING**

SLOW-ROAST BEEF BRISKET WITH JACKETS
SERVES 4

This is an underrated and good-value cut of beef. Slow cooking gives you lovely tender meat and means there is less for you to do. A perfect weekend dinner.

1 tbsp vegetable oil
1 onion, quartered
2 carrots, cut into chunks
4 celery sticks,
    cut into chunks
4 cloves garlic, roughly
    chopped
1kg boned, rolled
    beef brisket
500ml beef stock
    (fresh or made using
    1 low-salt stock cube)
1 × 400g tin chopped
    tomatoes
15g fresh thyme, chopped
4 large baking potatoes
Black pepper

1 Preheat the oven to 160°C/Fan 140°C.

2 Heat the oil in a large, heavy-based casserole dish that has a lid over a medium heat. Add the onion, carrots, celery and garlic and sauté for 5 minutes.

3 Place the beef in the dish and sear it for 2 minutes on each side until browned.

4 Stir in the stock, tomatoes and thyme and season with black pepper.

5 Cover the dish with a lid and cook in the oven for 4 hours, until the beef is very tender. Halfway through the cooking time, place the potatoes in the oven and cook alongside the beef.

6 Remove the dish from the oven and shred the beef using two forks.

7 Serve the shredded beef and vegetables with the baked potatoes and the sauce spooned over the top, alongside some steamed vegetables or a salad.

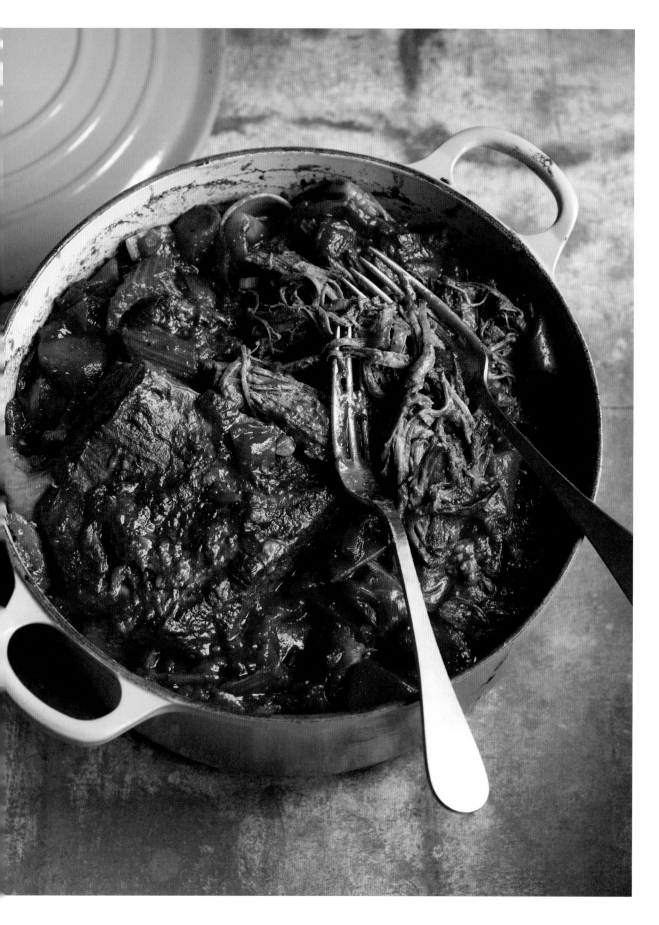

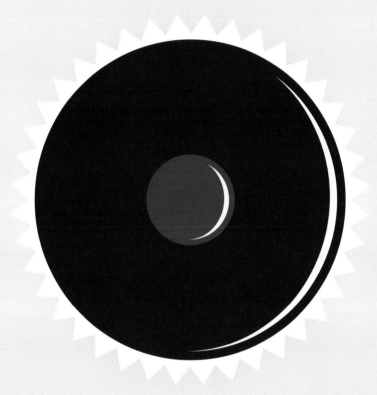

PUDDING

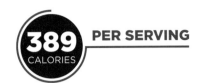 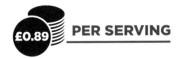

BERRY & APPLE CRUMBLE
SERVES 4

This is a simple crumble recipe that is great for a weekend pudding. It uses no flour and less butter than a typical recipe so it's a good way to enjoy something sweet without the extra calories.

3 apples, cored and
   chopped
1 tsp ground cinnamon
2 tbsp honey
150g porridge oats
50g ground almonds
35g unsalted butter, diced
400g frozen berries

1 Preheat the oven to 180°C/Fan 160°C.

2 Place the apples in a medium-sized crumble dish, sprinkle with the cinnamon and drizzle with 1 tablespoon of the honey. Add 2 tablespoons of water and bake in the oven for 20 minutes.

3 Meanwhile, put the oats, ground almonds and remaining honey into a bowl. Add the butter and rub well with your fingertips until you have a crumbly mixture. You could do this step in a food processor.

4 Add the frozen berries to the dish with the apples and scatter the crumble topping over the fruit. Bake in the oven for 35 minutes, until the top is golden and the fruit is bubbling below.

5 Serve with Greek yoghurt, if your calorie allowance permits.

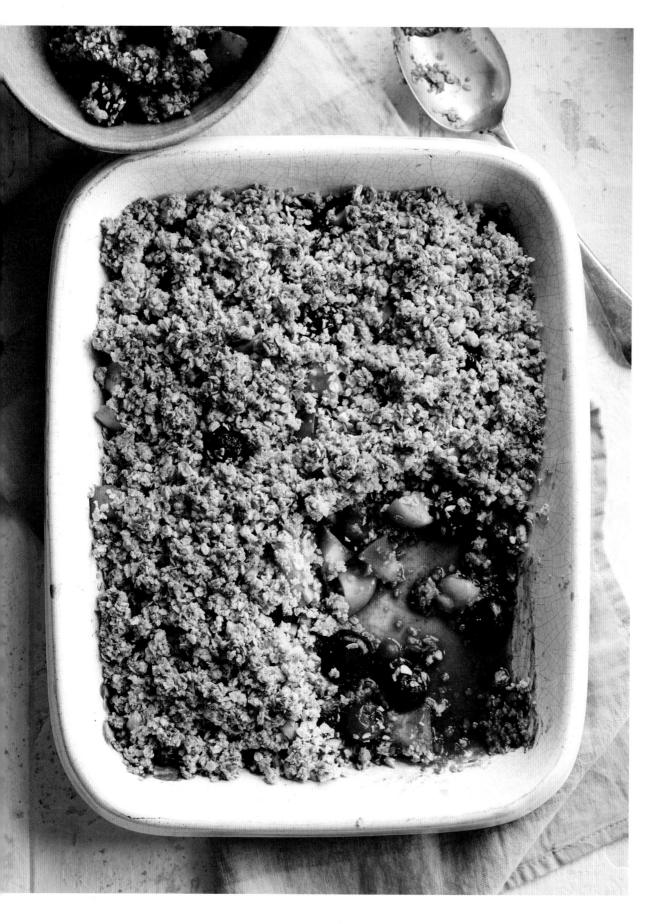

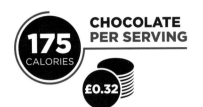

CHOCOLATE
PER SERVING
175 CALORIES
£0.32

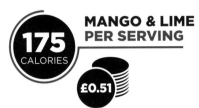

MANGO & LIME
PER SERVING
175 CALORIES
£0.51

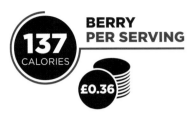

BERRY
PER SERVING
137 CALORIES
£0.36

INSTANT BANANA ICE CREAM THREE WAYS
SERVES 4

This is genius! The semi-thawed banana (once blitzed) gives a really creamy texture, similar to ice cream but without the calories. Keep a stash of peeled bananas in the freezer and you can whip these up in minutes.

CHOCOLATE
6 ripe bananas,
   peeled and frozen
2 tbsp cocoa powder
2 tsp honey

MANGO & LIME
4 ripe bananas,
   peeled and frozen
200g frozen chopped mango
75g natural yoghurt
Zest and juice of 1 lime
2 tsp honey

BERRY
4 ripe bananas,
   peeled and frozen
150g frozen berries
75g natural yoghurt

1 Whichever flavour you are making, place all of the ingredients in a food processor and pulse until just smooth.

2 Serve straight away or keep in the freezer for up to 40 minutes (after which it will start to freeze solid).

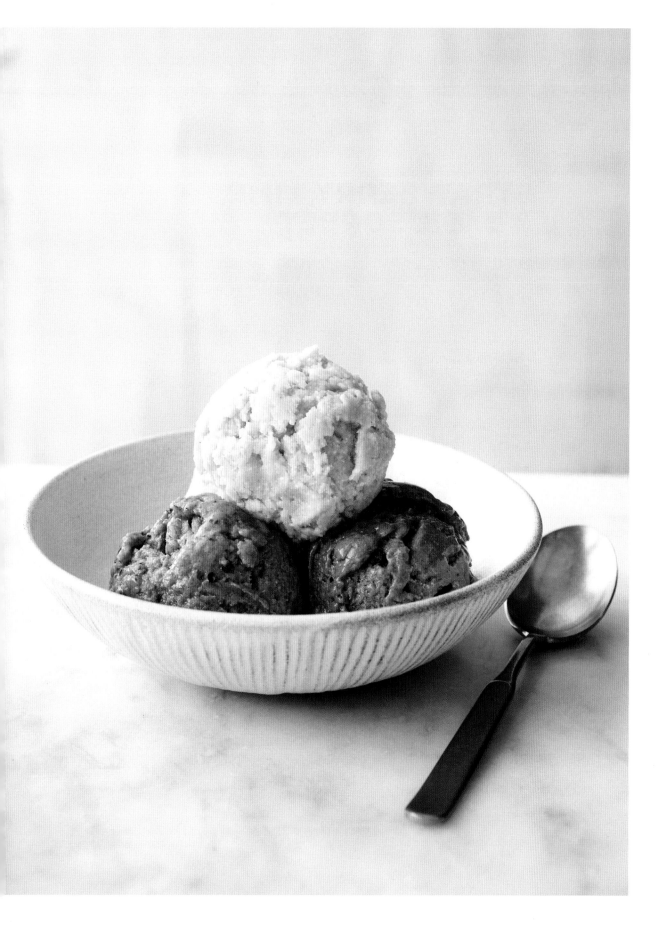

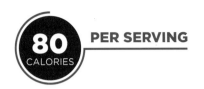

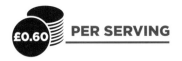 £0.60 **PER SERVING**

STRAWBERRY, LIME & BASIL SORBET
SERVES 4

A lovely, fresh and summery combination, this light pudding is for when you want something sweet but don't want to pile on the pounds.

550g fresh or frozen
   strawberries, stalks
   removed
Zest and juice of 1 lime
10g fresh basil
1 tbsp honey or maple
   syrup

1 If using frozen strawberries, remove them from the freezer and place in a bowl in the microwave for 3 minutes on high. This will help them blend more easily.

2 Place the strawberries in a food processor with all the remaining ingredients and whizz until just smooth. If using frozen strawberries, it will be a sorbet-like consistency and you can serve it straight away. Otherwise, spoon the mixture into an airtight container and return to the freezer.

3 After 30 minutes, remove from the freezer and mix with a fork to break up the crystals – this will ensure it freezes evenly. Return to the freezer for a further hour before serving.

4 Remove the sorbet from the freezer about 15–20 minutes before serving to give it time to soften enough to scoop and eat.

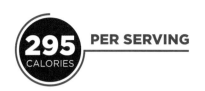
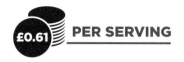

ROAST PINEAPPLE WITH ALMONDS & CRÈME FRAÎCHE
SERVES 4

This is a delicious, fruit-based, low-calorie pudding that is good enough to serve to guests too.

1 pineapple
50g light brown sugar
35g flaked almonds
100g half-fat crème fraîche
1 tsp vanilla essence
Zest of 1 lime

1 Preheat the oven to 200°C/Fan 180°C and line a baking tray with a large sheet of foil, making sure there is enough overhang to wrap the pineapple up into a parcel.

2 Peel the pineapple, slice it in half lengthways and cut into 1cm-thick slices. Place the slices on the foil.

3 Measure the brown sugar into a saucepan, add 3 tablespoons of water and place over a medium heat. Let it bubble for 1 minute until you have a thick syrup. Pour the syrup over the pineapple, then fold the overhanging foil over the pineapple. Scrunch the edges together to create a sealed parcel and bake in the oven for 30 minutes.

4 Remove the pineapple from the oven and open the top of the foil parcel so the pineapple pieces are no longer covered. Turn the temperature up to 220°C/Fan 200°C and return to the oven for a further 15 minutes until starting to brown.

5 Toast the almonds in a dry pan over a low heat until just brown on each side – be careful as they burn easily. Mix the crème fraîche with the vanilla.

6 Serve the pineapple hot from the oven, sprinkled with the toasted almonds and lime zest, with the vanilla crème fraîche on the side.

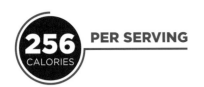 **PER SERVING**

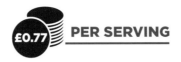 **PER SERVING**

FROZEN BERRIES WITH DARK CHOCOLATE SAUCE
SERVES 4

This is a very simple but delicious pudding. Perfect for entertaining.

300ml single cream
100g dark chocolate,
    chopped
400g mixed frozen berries

1 Heat the single cream in a small pan over a low heat until it just comes to the boil. Remove from the heat and stir in the chopped dark chocolate until it has melted.

2 Divide the berries between four bowls and pour over the hot chocolate sauce to serve.

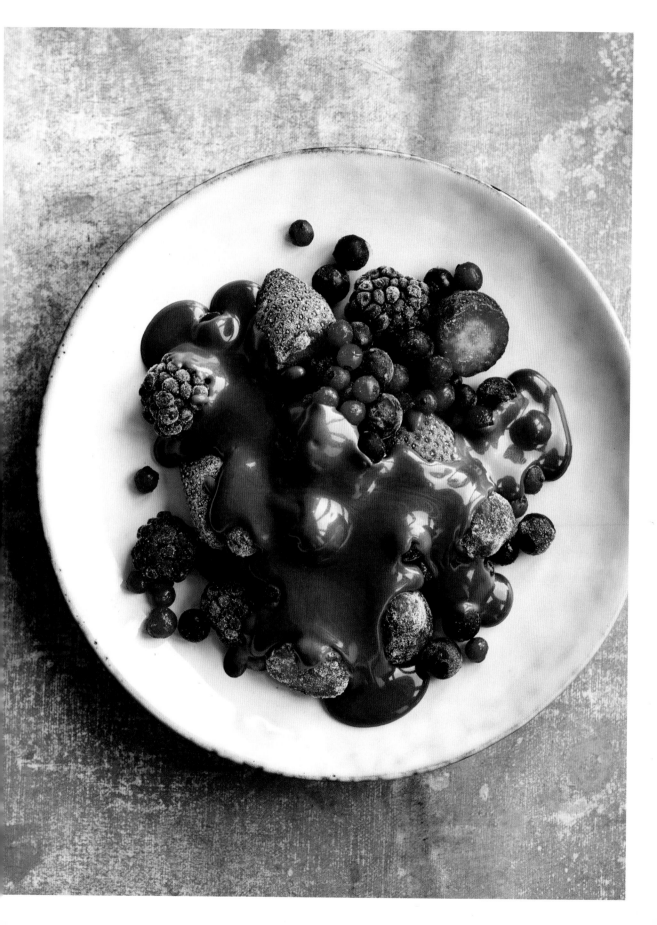

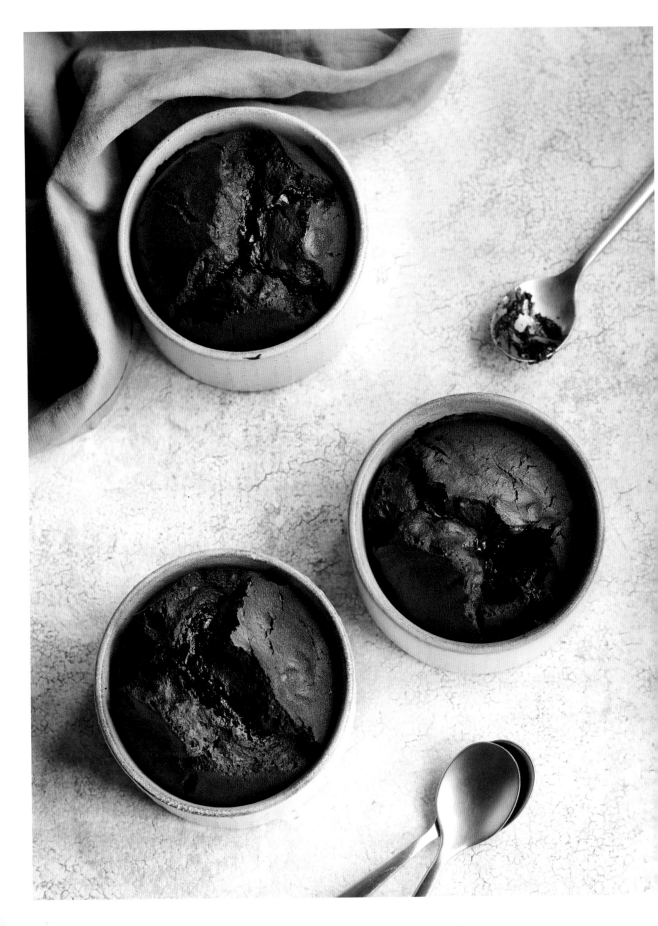

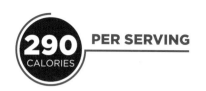 **PER SERVING**

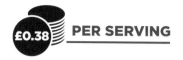 **PER SERVING**

GOOEY DARK CHOCOLATE POTS
SERVES 6

It's not a good idea to eat these regularly when you're trying to lose weight, but everyone needs a chocolatey treat every now and again and these are less calorific than most. Knowing that you have these up your sleeve to enjoy on a special occasion will mean you're less likely to fall off the diet wagon. These freeze really well, too. Increase the cooking time to 16 minutes and you can cook them straight from the freezer.

100g unsalted butter
150g dark chocolate,
   broken into pieces
4 eggs
75g caster sugar
50g self-raising flour
15g cocoa powder

1 Preheat the oven to 220°C/Fan 200°C.

2 Melt the butter and chocolate in a small pan over a low heat, stirring to ensure it doesn't catch. Remove from the heat and leave to cool a little.

3 Meanwhile, combine the eggs and sugar in a large bowl. Pour in the cooled chocolate and butter mixture and stir gently until just combined.

4 Sift the flour and cocoa powder into the bowl and fold through carefully until combined.

5 Spoon the mixture into six ramekins and bake in the oven for 10–12 minutes, until cooked on the outside but still soft and gooey in the middle.

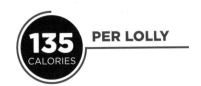

PER LOLLY

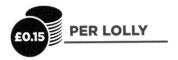

PER LOLLY

CHOCOLATE BANANA LOLLIES
MAKES 9 LOLLIES

This is a fun snack or pudding to make with little ones. Bananas have a lovely creamy texture when frozen. Feel free to mix up the toppings – use different nuts or try coating with freeze-dried raspberry pieces.

3 large bananas,
  each cut into three
75g dark chocolate
20g hazelnuts, chopped
  and toasted

1 Line a baking tray with baking parchment. You will need 9 lolly sticks or wooden skewers.

2 Insert a lolly stick or skewer into one end of each of the banana pieces and lay them on the tray. Place in the freezer for 2 hours or more until frozen.

3 To melt the chocolate, break it into a heatproof bowl and either place the bowl over a pan of barely simmering water, stirring occasionally, or place in the microwave and cook on low power so that it doesn't burn.

4 Holding the frozen bananas by the sticks or skewers, dip each one into the melted chocolate – you want to cover about half the banana.

5 Place the bananas back on the baking tray and sprinkle each one with chopped hazelnuts. Return to the freezer for at least another 30 minutes before serving. The bananas will keep in the freezer for up to a week if placed in an airtight container.

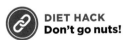

DIET HACK
Don't go nuts!

They seem like a good snack and are packed with nutrients but they are also packed with calories. A 25g portion of nuts (almonds, brazils or walnuts) comes in at around 125–150 calories. Try rice cakes or crunchy vegetable sticks instead. Be careful with nut allergies – especially with children.

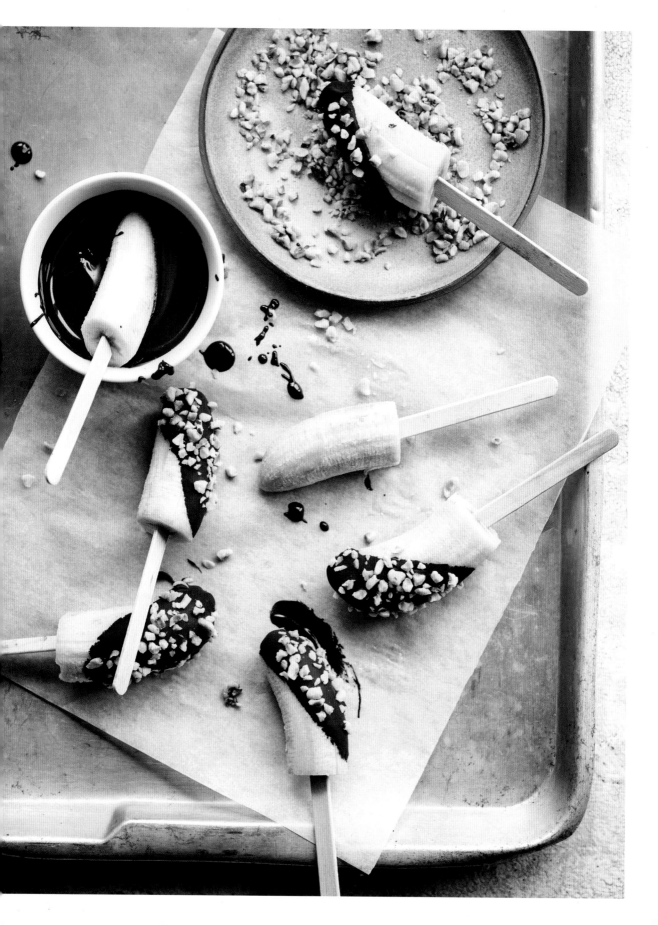

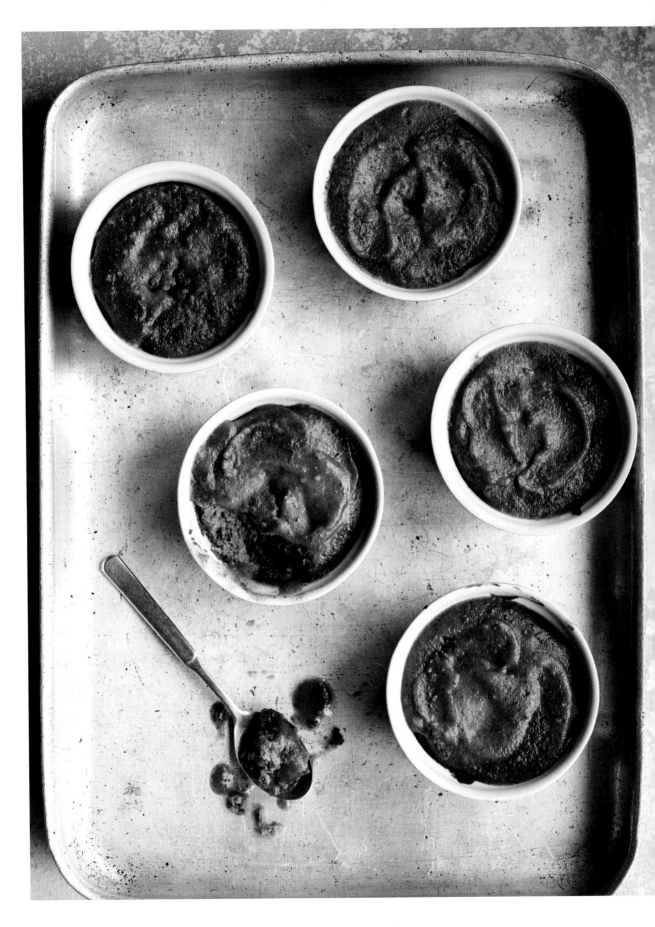

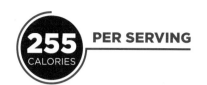 **255** CALORIES **PER SERVING**

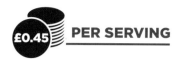 £0.45 **PER SERVING**

STICKY TOFFEE PUDDING WITH SALTED CARAMEL SAUCE
SERVES 6

Everyone needs a pudding once in a while and it's better to make it slightly lower cal but still delicious. Serve these in ramekins or one big dish.

For the puddings
175g pitted dates
150ml boiling water
50ml vegetable oil
2 tbsp maple syrup
2 eggs, separated
75g self-raising flour

For the sauce
50g pitted dates
75ml boiling water
1 tbsp unsalted butter
1 tbsp maple syrup
Pinch of sea salt

1 Preheat the oven to 200°C/Fan 180°C and grease 6 ramekins or 1 medium-sized ovenproof dish.

2 To make the puddings, place the dates in a heatproof bowl with the boiling water, cover with a plate and leave to soak for 10–15 minutes.

3 Pour the dates and their water into a food processor and whizz into a paste.

4 Place the date mixture, oil and maple syrup in a large bowl with the egg yolks and mix well. Sift in the flour and combine. Beat the egg whites until stiff peaks form. Fold the egg whites into the date mixture then spoon into the ramekins or dish. Bake in the oven for 20 minutes if using ramekins or 30–35 minutes if using one dish.

5 Meanwhile, to make the sauce, place the dates in a heatproof bowl with the boiling water and leave to soak for 10–15 minutes. Pour the dates and their water into a food processor and whizz into a paste.

6 Melt the butter in a small saucepan over a medium heat, add the maple syrup, a pinch of sea salt and the date paste and mix well.

7 Remove the puddings from the oven and serve with the sauce poured over the top.

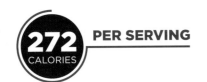 **PER SERVING**

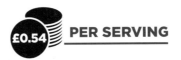 **PER SERVING**

CINNAMON & HONEY BAKED APPLES
SERVES 4

A delicious pudding packed full of zesty, warming flavours; it is quick and easy to make. Prepare the apples earlier in the day or the day before and bake them when you're ready.

4 eating apples, kept whole but cores removed
2 tsp ground cinnamon
2 tbsp honey
Zest of 1 orange
2 tbsp raisins
50g flaked almonds
25g unsalted butter

1 Preheat the oven to 200°C/Fan 180°C.

2 Score around the circumference of each apple with a small knife, just piercing the skin but not cutting too far into the flesh (this stops the apples exploding in the oven).

3 Mix the cinnamon, honey, orange zest, raisins and almonds together in a small bowl.

4 Place the apples in an ovenproof dish and spoon the raisin and almond mixture into the cored centre of each apple, pushing it down with a teaspoon. Top each apple with a small knob of butter and bake in the oven for approximately 35–40 minutes, or until golden and soft.

5 Leave to cool for 5 minutes before serving with a small spoonful of Greek yoghurt.

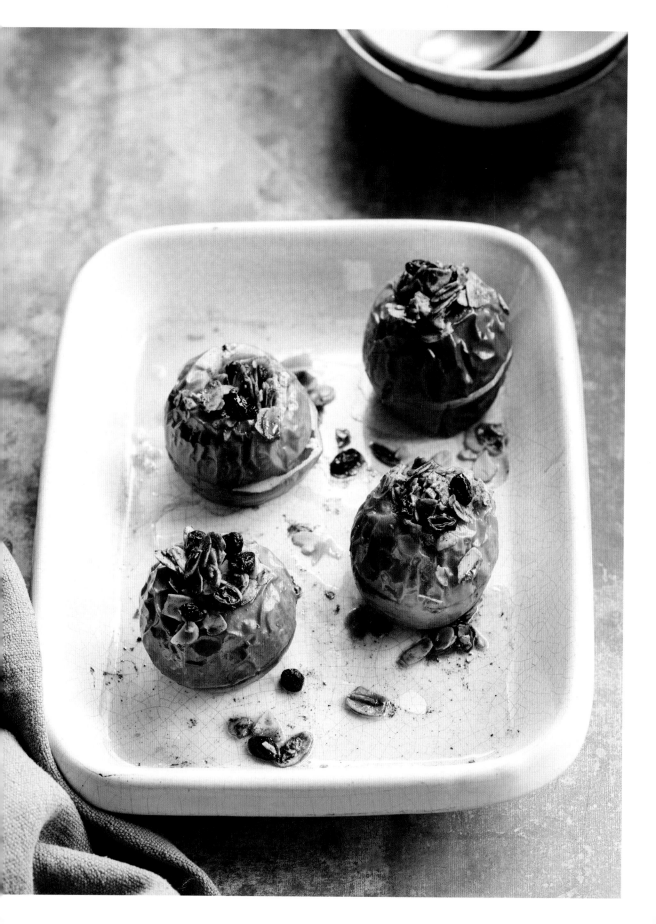

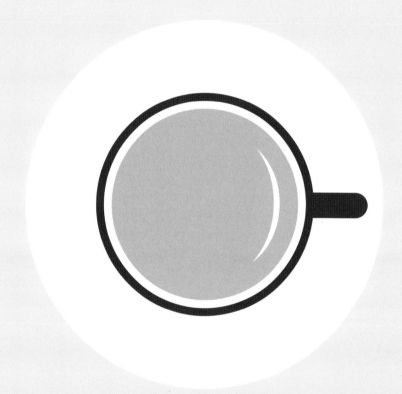

SNACKS & DRINKS

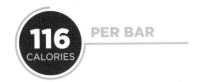 **116 CALORIES** PER BAR

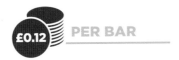 **£0.12** PER BAR

SAVOURY CHEESE, OAT & NUT BARS
MAKES 18 BARS

These savoury bars are perfect for when you would usually reach for some crisps. These also freeze well – make a batch, keep them in the freezer and you can defrost them individually as you need them. Make sure you let them cool completely in the tin before removing them or they will crumble.

150g porridge oats
100g carrot, grated
75g mixed nuts, finely chopped (I do this by whizzing them in a food processor)
75g Cheddar, grated
100g unsalted butter, melted
1 tsp mustard powder

1 Preheat the oven to 200°C/Fan 180°C and line a square 23cm baking tin.

2 Combine all of the ingredients in a large bowl and mix well.

3 Spoon the mixture into the prepared tin, press it down with the back of a spoon to level. Bake in the oven for 25 minutes until golden brown.

4 Leave to cool completely in the tin.

5 Turn out on to a board and cut into 18 bars.

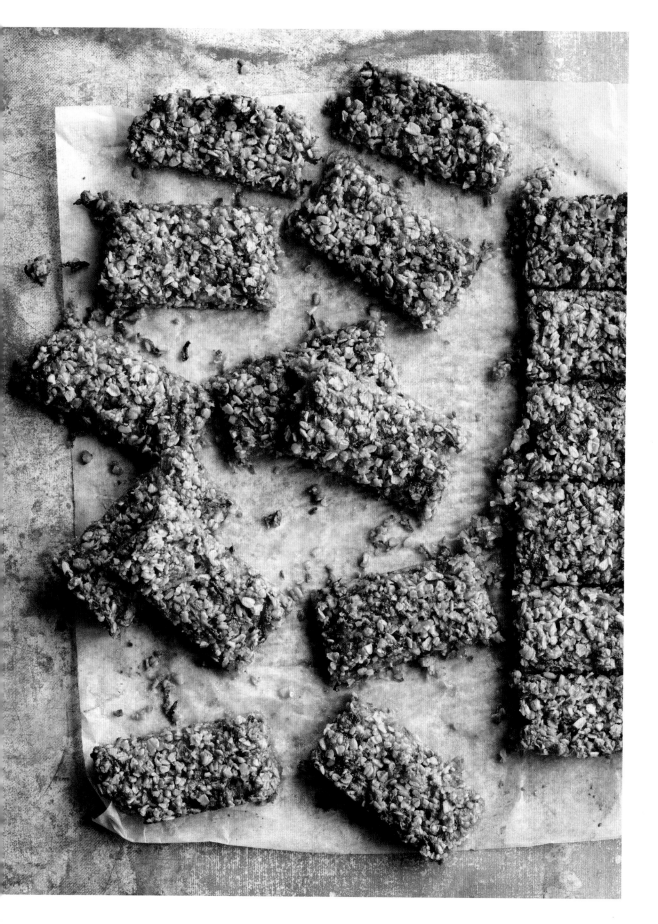

DIPS THREE WAYS

Dips are a good thing to have in the fridge for snacking during the week.

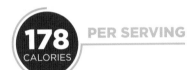 **PER SERVING**

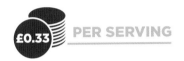 **PER SERVING**

1 CHICKPEA & PESTO DIP
SERVES 6 AS A SNACK

This is a delicious snack to serve with raw vegetable batons or spread on to oatcakes or toasted rye bread. It is nice served as a light starter and would also work really well as a sandwich filler; try it in a Spinach Wrap (see page 88).

1 × 400g tin chickpeas,
   drained
30g fresh basil
2 tbsp olive oil
15g Parmesan, grated
1 clove garlic
Zest of 1 lemon
Pinch of black pepper

1 Put all of the ingredients in a food processor with 200ml water and whizz until smooth.

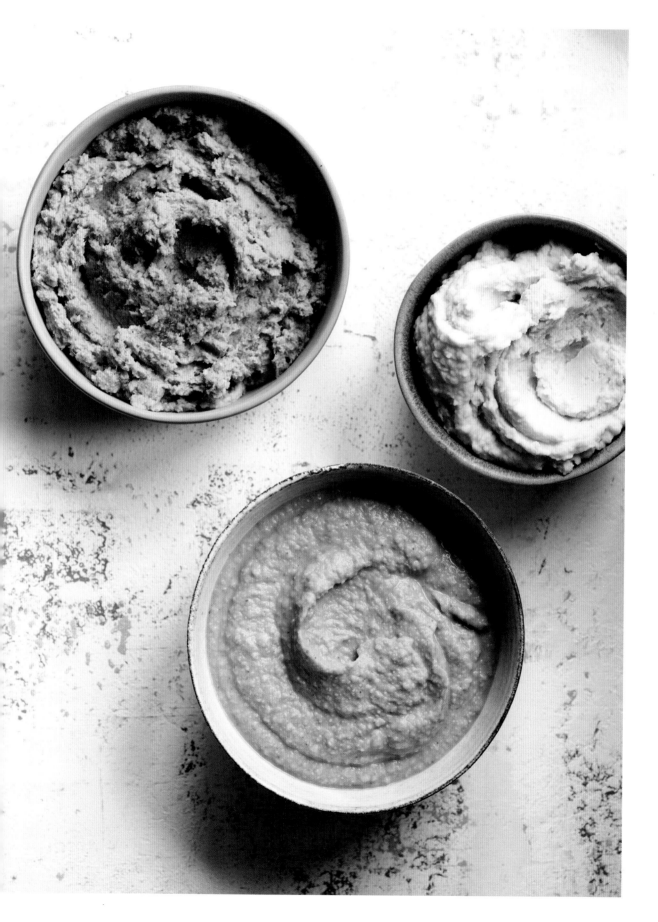

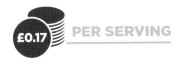

103 CALORIES PER SERVING

£0.17 PER SERVING

2 BUTTERBEAN LEMON DIP
SERVES 6 AS A SNACK

This is a great protein-packed dip, perfect for snacking or to serve before a dinner party. It's also really delicious spread on toast and topped with some veggies or smoked salmon as a quick lunch.

1 × 400g tin butterbeans, drained
1 clove garlic
2 tbsp olive oil
1 tbsp tahini
Zest and juice of 1 lemon
Pinch of black pepper

1 Place all the ingredients together in a food processor with 3 tablespoons of water and whizz until well blended.

2 Serve in a small bowl with a selection of raw vegetable crudités.

102 CALORIES PER SERVING

£0.33 PER SERVING

3 SMOKED MACKEREL PATÉ
SERVES 6 AS A SNACK

Make a batch at the weekend and keep it in an airtight container in the fridge to spread on oatcakes or serve with crudités during the week.

1 smoked mackerel fillet, skin removed
1 × 400g tin butterbeans, drained
2 tsp smoked paprika
Juice of 1 lemon
2 tbsp natural yoghurt
Pinch of black pepper

1 Put all of the ingredients in a food processor and whizz until smooth.

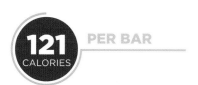
121 CALORIES | PER BAR

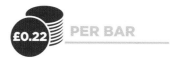
£0.22 | PER BAR

FRUITY FLAPJACK BITES
MAKES 18 BARS

These little bites are a great snack to have in the cupboard (or freezer) for when sweet cravings hit. Keep them in the freezer and defrost them individually, if having the whole lot out is too tempting! They're a great addition to a packed lunch.

200g dried apricots
100ml boiling water
50g peanut butter
1 tbsp honey
150g porridge oats
1 tbsp vegetable oil
100g flaked almonds

1 Preheat the oven to 200°C/Fan 180°C and line a baking tray (approx. 33 × 23cm) with baking parchment.

2 Put the apricots, water and peanut butter into a food processor and whizz. Add the remaining ingredients and pulse a couple of times so the oats are still chunky but combined.

3 Spoon the mixture into the lined baking tray and flatten evenly with the back of the spoon. Bake in the oven for 15 minutes until firm and golden.

4 Remove from the oven and leave to cool slightly in the tin for 10–15 minutes, then loosen the edges with a knife and cut into 18 bars. Remove from the tin and leave to cool completely on a wire rack.

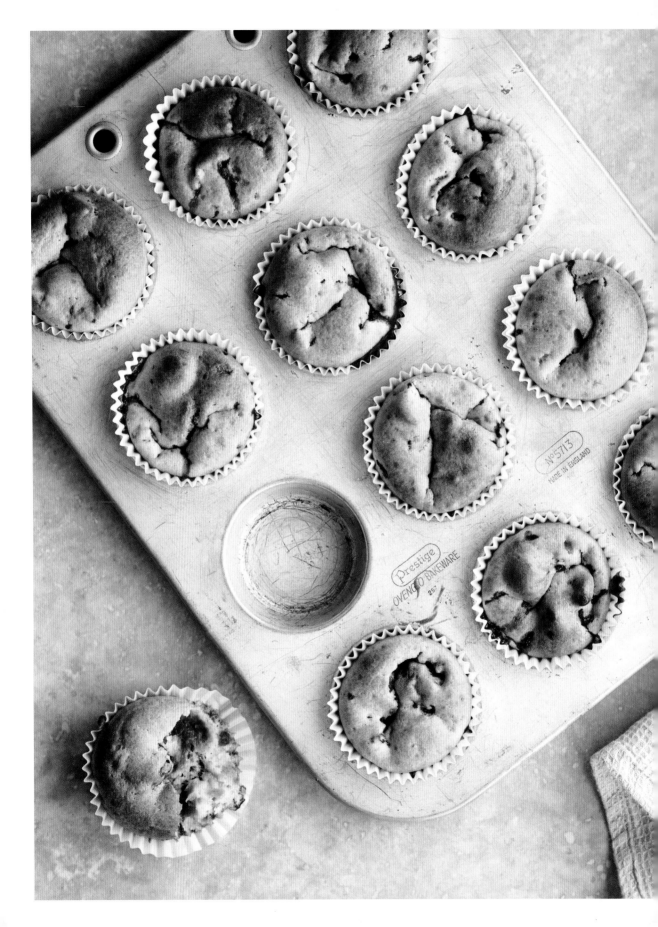

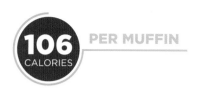
106 CALORIES PER MUFFIN

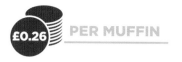
£0.26 PER MUFFIN

LEMON & RASPBERRY MINI MUFFINS
MAKES 12 MUFFINS

It's a great idea to have a low-cal cake recipe up your sleeve. Whip up a batch of these at the weekend to satisfy those afternoon cravings. These freeze well, too, and are a hit with little ones.

2 eggs
2 tbsp honey
50ml vegetable oil
150g natural yoghurt
125g plain flour
½ tsp baking powder
Zest of 1 lemon
100g raspberries

1 Preheat the oven to 180°C/Fan 160°C and place 12 fairy cake cases in a muffin tin.

2 Mix the eggs, honey, oil and yoghurt together in a small bowl.

3 Tip the flour, baking powder and lemon zest into a large bowl, then add the wet ingredients to the dry and combine with a fork. Do not over mix or the muffins will be a little tough. Add the raspberries and mix briefly until combined.

4 Spoon the mixture into the cases and bake for 20–25 minutes or until risen, cooked through and golden brown.

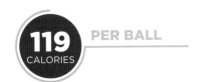
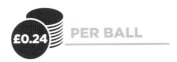

COCONUT CHOCOLATE ORANGE ENERGY BALL BITES
MAKES 10 BALLS

These are perfect for an afternoon pick-me-up. Keep one in your bag for when those sugar cravings hit after lunch. They also freeze well so you can defrost them individually as you need them.

75g dates
50g porridge oats
50g unsalted peanuts
1 tbsp cocoa powder
Zest and juice of 1 orange
110g desiccated coconut
1 tbsp boiling water

1 Place the dates in a heatproof bowl, cover with boiling water and set aside for 5–10 minutes until soft.

2 Drain any excess water from the dates and place in a food processor with the oats, peanuts, cocoa powder and orange zest and juice. Add 75g of the desiccated coconut and the boiling water. Whizz until fully combined.

3 With wet hands, roll the mixture into balls, approximately the size of a golf ball, and then roll in the remaining desiccated coconut until evenly coated.

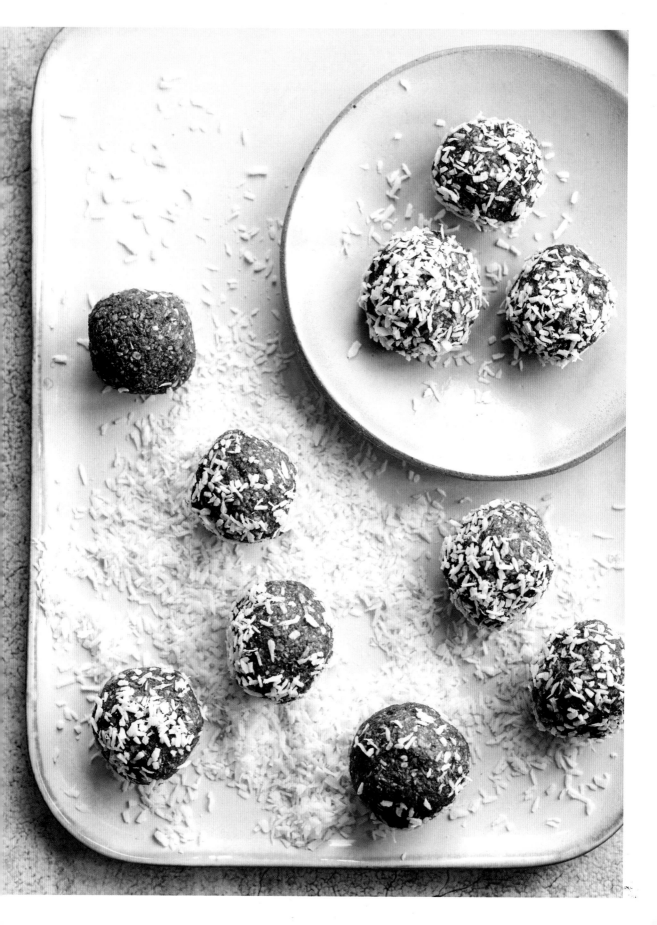

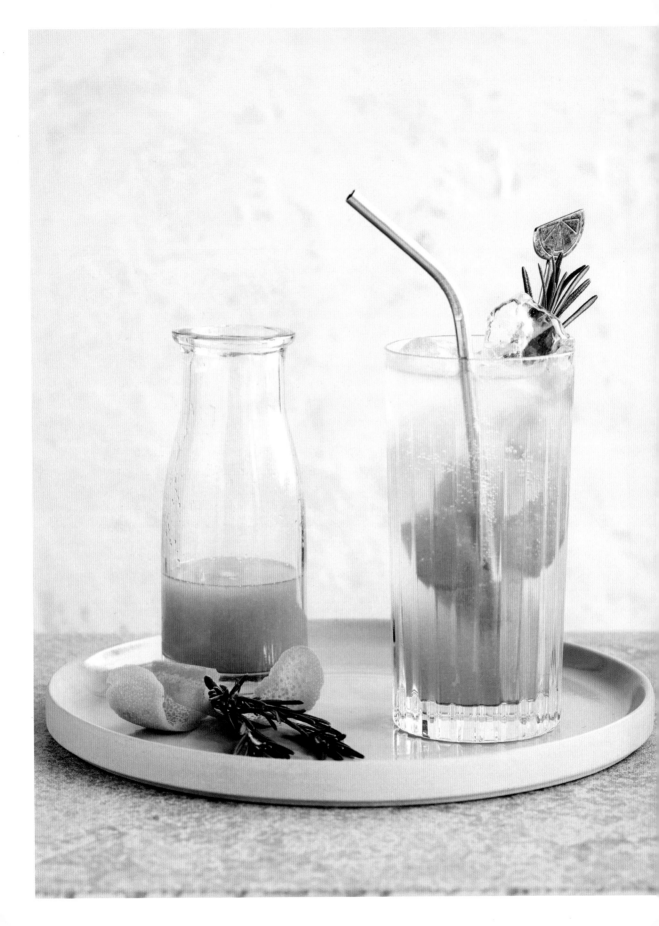

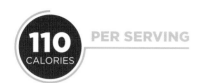 **PER SERVING**

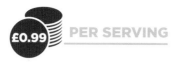 **PER SERVING**

ZESTY CITRUS GIN & TONIC
SERVES 2

A vibrant twist on the classic gin and tonic. Always remember to drink sensibly. UK guidelines are that you should not drink more than 14 units of alcohol per week. Of course, if you are looking to lose weight you will need to keep an eye on the calorie count in alcoholic drinks, as well.

1 grapefruit
1 orange
4 ice cubes
50ml gin
250ml tonic
2 sprigs rosemary

1 Peel a couple of strips each of grapefruit and orange rind and place them in two glasses with the ice cubes.

2 Cut the grapefruit and orange in half and squeeze half of each fruit into a small bowl or jug. Divide this citrus juice between the glasses. Cut the remaining fruit halves into wedges and place a couple pieces of each fruit into each glass.

3 Divide the gin between the glasses then top up with the tonic.

4 Finally, add a rosemary sprig to each glass and serve.

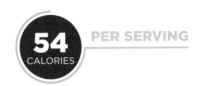
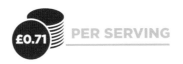
VODKA & ELDERFLOWER FIZZ
SERVES 2

A good cocktail to have up your sleeve for those evenings when you want an alcoholic treat but don't want to blow the calories. Perfect for a summer barbecue. Always remember to drink sensibly. UK guidelines are that you should not drink more than 14 units of alcohol per week. Of course, if you are looking to lose weight you will need to keep an eye on the calorie count in alcoholic drinks, as well. (Also pictured is **Pomegranate, Mint & Lime Mocktail** – in the right-hand glass – on page 202.)

Zest of 1 lemon
4 ice cubes
50ml vodka
2 tsp elderflower cordial
250ml soda water

1 Divide the lemon zest, ice cubes and vodka between two glasses.

2 Add a teaspoon of elderflower cordial to each glass then top with the soda water to serve.

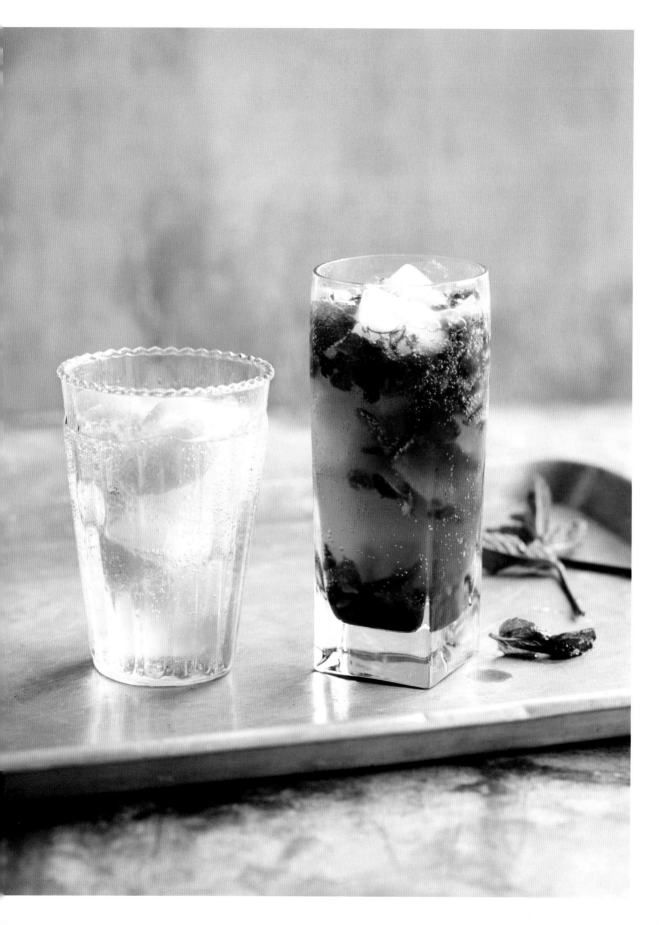

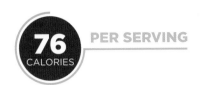

76 CALORIES — PER SERVING

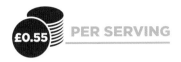

£0.55 — PER SERVING

POMEGRANATE, MINT & LIME MOCKTAIL
SERVES 2

An impressive drink to serve up to friends and family. Make this in individual glasses or in a big jug to put in the middle of the table.

4 sprigs mint, leaves picked
3 tbsp pomegranate seeds
Juice of 1 lime
4 ice cubes
Soda water

1 Crush the mint leaves and pomegranate seeds in a pestle and mortar and divide between two glasses.

2 Divide the lime juice between the glasses and add the ice. Top up with soda water and give it a quick stir before serving.

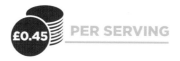
GINGER, LEMON & TURMERIC TEA

SERVES 2

This is a really good alternative to tea or coffee. Delicious served after dinner and, as it's packed with antibacterial ingredients, is perfect for the flu season.

Juice of 1 lemon
1 thumb-sized piece of fresh root ginger, peeled and finely sliced, or pounded in a pestle and mortar for a stronger flavour
1 tsp ground turmeric
500ml boiling water

1 Place all of the ingredients into a teapot and leave to brew for 5 minutes.

2 Pour the tea through a strainer into two mugs to serve.

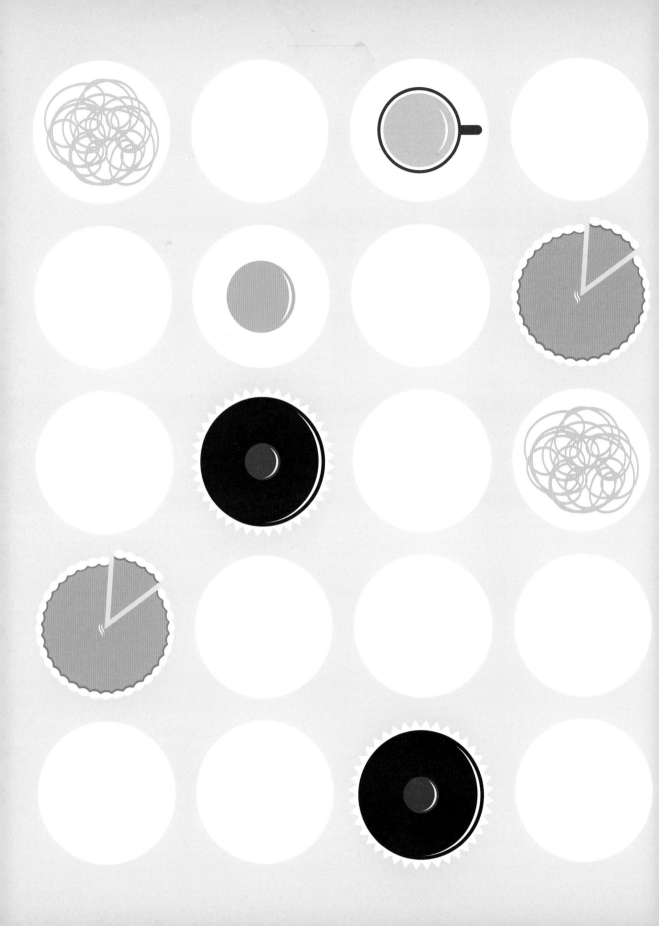

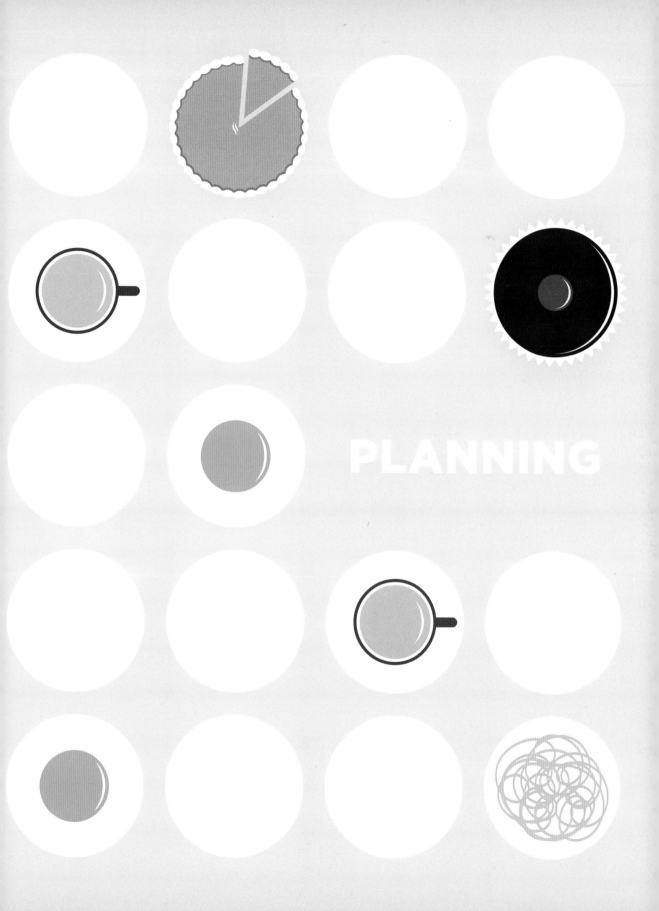

PLANNING

STORE CUPBOARD

Stocking your kitchen with some essentials will make it much easier to create a home-cooked meal, even when you don't have much in the fridge. It may look like a lot, but once you've stocked your store cupboard, the majority of the ingredients will last for a while and add heaps of flavour to many dishes. Look around the supermarkets to find the cheapest brands to save money.

- Olive oil
- Vegetable oil
- Sesame oil (excellent for adding flavour to Asian recipes – a little goes a long way)
- Vinegar (balsamic, cider and/ or white wine)
- Low-salt soy sauce
- Honey
- Peanut butter
- Dijon mustard
- Fish sauce (great for adding depth of flavour to Asian dishes and dressings)
- Miso paste (full of protein so great for non-meat eaters and readily available)
- Lentils
- Brown rice
- Dried pasta
- Dried noodles
- Tinned tomatoes
- Tinned sweetcorn

- Tinned coconut milk
- Salt & black pepper
- Garam masala
- Ground turmeric
- Ground cinnamon
- Ground coriander
- Cinnamon sticks
- Chinese 5-spice
- Dried oregano
- Smoked paprika
- Nutmeg
- Fennel seeds
- Chilli flakes
- Low-salt stock cubes (chicken, beef and/or vegetable)
- Self-raising flour
- Plain flour
- Cornflour
- Cocoa powder
- Vanilla extract

KITCHEN EQUIPMENT

Ensuring you have a well-equipped kitchen will make cooking so much easier and more enjoyable. This isn't about spending a fortune on all the bells and whistles. You really can make the majority of these recipes with some basic knives, chopping boards and pots and pans.

Here's our list of realistic equipment if you're starting from scratch or want a check list:

- Sharp knives & a knife sharpener (this really extends the life of your knives and keeps them sharp)
- Vegetable peeler
- A couple of wooden spoons
- Potato masher
- Chopping boards
- Non-stick frying pan & saucepans
- Baking tray & ovenproof ceramic dishes
- Whisk

- Colander
- Sieve
- Grater
- Zester
- Pestle and mortar
- Mixing bowl
- Kitchen scales
- Food processor (you can pick one up for around £24.99, so it needn't be a big expense! If you spend more, remember it's an investment and will last for years)

THE FOUR-WEEK MEAL PLANNER

This delicious four-week meal planner will help you to count calories without skimping on flavour or fun. Each recipe is calorie counted with a total given for each day, too. The ingredients for these breakfast, lunch and dinner recipes are all reasonably priced and easy to find at your local supermarket. It couldn't be simpler!

We appreciate everyone's lifestyle and BMI is different, so there are recipes for snacks, too – you can choose which snacks to add to your daily plan, making sure you stay within your personal calorie allowance for successful weight loss (for most men this is no more than 1,900 kcals per day and for most women no more than 1,400 kcals per day).

Personally, I need to have treats, so there are low-cal recipes for puddings, too. Perhaps your calorie count will allow for one of these midweek? Or at the weekend as well? Perhaps you fancy a treat in the form of a tipple instead? The calorie counts are provided for all of the drinks, so you can work it out for yourself easily, while still staying on track.

Finally, I have included an 'at a glance' calorie counter to remind you of the impact some of your normal sides, go-to snacks and drinks can have on your diet.

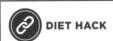 **DIET HACK**

Chew gum not crisps!
Chewing sugar-free gum, especially in the afternoon, can help you feel satisfied and less likely to snack. Plus it's good for your teeth!

CALORIE COUNTS FOR TREATS

Snacks	Kcals per serving
Smoked Mackerel Paté	102
Butterbean Lemon Dip	103
Lemon & Raspberry Mini Muffins	106
Savoury Cheese, Oat & Nut Bars	116
Coconut Chocolate Orange Energy Ball Bites	119
Fruity Flapjack Bites	121
Chickpeas & Pesto Dip	178

Drinks	Kcals per serving
Ginger, Lemon & Turmeric Tea	21
Vodka & Elderflower Fizz	54
Pomegranate, Mint & Lime Mocktail	76
Zesty Citrus Gin & Tonic	110

Puddings	Kcals per serving
Strawberry, Lime & Basil Sorbet	80
Chocolate Banana Lollies	135
Berry Banana Ice Cream	137
Chocolate Banana Ice Cream	175
Mango & Lime Banana Ice Cream	175
Sticky Toffee Pudding with Salted Caramel Sauce	255
Frozen Berries with Dark Chocolate Sauce	256
Cinnamon & Honey Baked Apples	272
Gooey Dark Chocolate Pots	290
Roast Pineapple with Almonds & Crème Fraîche	295
Berry & Apple Crumble	389

CALORIE COUNTS FOR SIDES

	Kcals
1 serving green salad	15
1 portion (80g) steamed greens	15
1 serving tomato salad	22
100g boiled new potatoes	75
100g cooked brown rice	111
100g cooked pasta	157
1 small (180g) baked potato	175

AT A GLANCE CALORIE COUNTER

	Kcals
1 digestive biscuit	71
2 small pears	100
1 banana	100
166g grapes	100
24g Cheddar	100
20g corn chips	100
2 oranges	100
175ml glass of wine (12% Strength)	126
25g portion of nuts	150
1 bowl of cornflakes with milk	172
1 slice of toast & butter	210
1 pint of beer (5% strength)	215
1 avocado	227
1 plain croissant	231

WEEK ONE MEAL PLANNER

	BREAKFAST	**LUNCH**	**DINNER**
MONDAY TOTAL 893 CALS	Banana & Cinnamon Porridge (page 56) 325 calories	Sunshine Soup (page 83) 129 calories	Easy Thai Green Curry (page 141) 439 calories
TUESDAY TOTAL 946 CALS	Green Smoothie (page 60) 151 calories	Filled Homemade Spinach Wraps (e.g. with vegetables and chicken) (page 88) 388 calories	Lentil & Tomato Bolognaise (page 134) 407 calories
WEDNESDAY TOTAL 775 CALS	Spiced Apple Overnight Oats (page 57) 256 calories	Egg, Cottage Cheese & Rocket Open Sandwich (page 82) 83 calories	Super Easy Fish Tray Bake (page 151) 436 calories
THURSDAY TOTAL 1124 CALS	Easy Fridge Raid Omelette (page 73) 236 calories	Rainbow Vegetable & Feta Salad (page 96) 556 calories	Turkey Meatballs with Tomato Sauce (page 136) 332 calories
FRIDAY TOTAL 1096 CALS	Quick Banana & Oat Pancakes (page 62) 309 calories	New Potato & Courgette Frittata (page 92) 225 calories	Easy Homemade Pizza (page 118) 562 calories
SATURDAY TOTAL 1229 CALS	One-dish Cooked Breakfast (page 77) 249 calories	Spinach & Feta Tart (page 95) 558 calories	Pork Chops with Roast Vegetable Ratatouille (page 159) 422 calories
SUNDAY TOTAL 1287 CALS	Mexican-style Eggs (page 68) 333 calories	Easy Sunday Roast Chicken with One-tray Vegetables (page 112) 515 calories	Spiced Bean & Lentil Chilli (page 126) 439 calories

WEEK ONE SHOPPING LIST

Fruit & Vegetables

2 apples

6 bananas

2 lemons

2 limes

3 avocados

450g cherry tomatoes

2 small cooked beetroot

1 cucumber

1 × bag salad leaves, e.g.
   rocket

2 spring onions

1 aubergine

1 butternut squash

12 carrots

200g chestnut
   mushrooms

6 courgettes

1 bulb of fennel

150g fresh spinach

400g green beans

200g mushrooms

350g parsnips

1kg new potatoes

4 red or orange peppers

500g sweet potatoes

10 onions

2 red onions

2 heads of garlic

1 red or green chilli

2.5cm piece of fresh
   root ginger

45g fresh basil

60g fresh coriander

15g fresh flat-leaf parsley

Dairy

350ml semi-skimmed
   milk

545g natural yoghurt

150g cottage cheese

325g feta

2 × 125g balls mozzarella

1 × 320g packet ready-
   rolled puff pastry

Meat & Fish

4 cod fillets

1 whole chicken
   (approx. 1.5kg)

4 skinless, boneless
   chicken thighs

400g turkey mince

4 rashers unsmoked
   back bacon

4 pork chops (bone-in)

250g beef mince

Frozen

485g frozen spinach

**Store cupboard staples
(bread, eggs, dried
goods)**

2 slices bread

27 eggs

300g brown rice

160g couscous

200g brown lentils

100g red lentils

250g porridge oats

320g wholewheat
   spaghetti

25g pine nuts

75g sundried tomatoes

400g tomato passata

1 × 400g tin black beans

1 × 400g tin kidney
   beans

6 × 400g tins tinned
   tomatoes

1 × 400ml tin coconut
   milk

50g capers

Shopping list quantities reflect the number of people the recipe is stated as serving.
Please refer to individual recipes and scale up or down depending on how many
people you are cooking for.

WEEK TWO MEAL PLANNER

	BREAKFAST	LUNCH	DINNER
MONDAY TOTAL **824** CALS	Oat, Berry & Coconut Smoothie (page 58) 325 calories	Creamy Roast Tomato & Basil Soup (page 85) 97 calories	Zingy Courgette Carbonara (page 156) 402 calories
TUESDAY TOTAL **1274** CALS	Spinach & Egg French Toast (page 64) 312 calories	Spiced Roast Chickpea & Cauliflower Salad (page 102) 445 calories	Teriyaki Beef & Pea Stir-fry (page 165) 517 calories
WEDNESDAY TOTAL **871** CALS	Egg, Bacon & Spinach Breakfast Muffins (page 70) 109 calories	DIY Instant Miso Veggie Soup Jars (page 87) 256 calories	Sausage Ragu with Brown Rice (page 160) 506 calories
THURSDAY TOTAL **758** CALS	Banana & Cinnamon Porridge (page 56) 325 calories	Creamy Cucumber & Smoked Salmon Open Sandwich (page 82) 108 calories	Sweet Potato, Chickpea & Spinach Curry (page 122) 325 calories
FRIDAY TOTAL **831** CALS	Egg, Bacon & Spinach Breakfast Muffins (page 70) 109 calories	Vietnamese Beef Salad (page 115) 375 calories	Aromatic Chicken & Rice Broth (page 135) 347 calories
SATURDAY TOTAL **1217** CALS	Sweetcorn Fritters with Poached Eggs (page 66) 364 calories	Minestrone with Pesto (page 86) 431 calories	Chinese Pork Noodles (page 154) 422 calories
SUNDAY TOTAL **1189** CALS	Green Smoothie (page 60) 151 calories	Vegetable Pad Thai (page 99) 411 calories	Slow-roast Beef Brisket with Jackets (page 166) 627 calories

WEEK TWO SHOPPING LIST

Fruit & Vegetables

2 bananas
2 lemons
5 limes
1 avocado
6 celery sticks
1 cucumber
1 Little Gem lettuce
200g radishes
125g salad leaves
2 bunches spring onions
1.6kg tomatoes
200g beansprouts
13 carrots
1 small cauliflower
5 courgettes
200g fresh spinach
150g green beans
300g any green
  vegetables
525g mushrooms
150g sugar snap peas
2 sweet potatoes
4 large baking potatoes
2 red chillies
4 onions
3 red onions
3 heads of garlic
10cm piece of fresh
  root ginger
45g fresh basil
15g fresh chives
45g fresh coriander
10g fresh dill
15g fresh mint
45g fresh flat-leaf parsley
15g fresh thyme
15g any soft fresh herbs

Dairy

2 tsp unsalted butter
200ml semi-skimmed milk
195g natural yoghurt
60g Parmesan

Meat & Fish

75g smoked salmon
1 whole chicken
  (approx. 1.4kg)
8 pork or chicken sausages
10 rashers unsmoked
  streaky bacon
500g lean pork mince
480g rump steak
1kg boned, rolled beef
  brisket

Frozen

175g frozen berries
400g frozen petits pois
  or frozen peas
405g frozen spinach

Store cupboard staples (bread, eggs, dried goods)

10 slices bread
24 eggs
725g brown rice
450g egg noodles
200g rice noodles
125g porridge oats
100g small dried pasta
  shapes (for soup)
200g wholewheat
  spaghetti
2 × 400ml tins coconut
  milk
1 × 400g tin cannellini
  beans
2 × 400g tins chickpeas
2 × 198g tins sweetcorn
3 × 400g tins tinned
  tomatoes
1 tsp fennel seeds
1 cinnamon stick
35g unsalted almonds
35g unsalted peanuts
25g peanut butter
60g miso paste

NB You will also need
200g cooked grains

Shopping list quantities reflect the number of people the recipe is stated as serving. Please refer to individual recipes and scale up or down depending on how many people you are cooking for.

WEEK THREE MEAL PLANNER

	BREAKFAST	LUNCH	DINNER
MONDAY TOTAL 840 CALS	Quick Mushroom & Tomato Breakfast Scramble (page 65) 199 calories	Rainbow Veg Stuffed Sweet Potatoes (page 100) 393 calories	Butternut Squash & Green Bean Tagine (page 125) 248 calories
TUESDAY TOTAL 1233 CALS	Chocolate Orange Porridge (page 54) 332 calories	Zingy Prawn & Noodle Salad Jar Shakers (page 106) 328 calories	Peri Peri Chicken with Crispy Potatoes (page 145) 573 calories
WEDNESDAY TOTAL 1075 CALS	Tropical Citrus Smoothie (page 61) 265 calories	Filled Homemade Spinach Wraps (e.g. with vegetables and chicken) (page 88) 388 calories	Salmon with Creamy Potato, Cucumber, Dill & Radish Salad (page 146) 422 calories
THURSDAY TOTAL 1031 CALS	Quick Banana & Oat Pancakes (page 62) 309 calories	Tomato, Basil & Butterbean Open Sandwich (page 80) 191 calories	Sweet Potato Gnocchi with Pesto (page 120) 531 calories
FRIDAY TOTAL 971 CALS	Easy Fridge Raid Omelette (page 73) 236 calories	DIY Instant Miso Veggie Soup Jars (page 87) 256 calories	Pearl Barley, Bacon & Kale Warmer (page 152) 479 calories
SATURDAY TOTAL 1150 CALS	One-dish Cooked Breakfast (page 77) 249 calories	Cheesy Mushroom, Avocado & Sweetcorn Quesadilla (page 91) 580 calories	Mushroom & Butterbean Burgers with Sweet Potato Wedges (page 131) 321 calories
SUNDAY TOTAL 1109 CALS	Vegetable Fritters with Garlic Roast Tomatoes (page 74) 228 calories	Spiced Turkey Mince & Avocado Lettuce Cups (page 109) 363 calories	Slow-cooked Lamb with Butterbean Mash (page 162) 518 calories

WEEK THREE SHOPPING LIST

Fruit & Vegetables

5 bananas

3 lemons

3 limes

3 oranges

4 avocados

750g cherry tomatoes

1 cucumber

6 Little Gem lettuces

150g radishes

2 bunches spring onions

175g tomatoes

9 carrots

500g butternut squash

5 courgettes

140g green beans

325g kale

675g mushrooms

6 Portobello mushrooms

500g new potatoes

800g potatoes

2 red peppers

9 sweet potatoes

350g any mixed
   vegetables

2 onions

3 red onions

3 heads of garlic

3 red chillies

45g fresh basil

75g fresh coriander

15g fresh dill

6 sprigs rosemary

15g fresh thyme

30g any soft fresh herbs

Dairy

2 tsp unsalted butter

350ml semi-skimmed
   milk

200ml almond milk
   (or any other dairy/
   non-dairy milk)

180g natural yoghurt

100g Cheddar

Parmesan

Meat & Fish

150g cooked king
   prawns

4 salmon fillets

4 chicken thighs

4 chicken drumsticks

500g turkey mince

12 rashers unsmoked
   back bacon

2kg shoulder of lamb

Frozen

135g frozen spinach

175g frozen tropical fruit

**Store cupboard staples
(bread, eggs, dried
goods)**

2 slices bread

4 wholemeal tortilla
   wraps

17 eggs

60g egg noodles

225g porridge oats

250g brown rice or
   couscous

300g pearl barley

300g quinoa

4 × 400g tins butter
   beans

2 × 198g tins sweetcorn

2 × 400g tins tinned
   tomatoes

50g unsalted almonds

60g tomato purée

45g miso paste

75g panko breadcrumbs

*NB You will also need
200g cooked grains*

Shopping list quantities reflect the number of people the recipe is stated as serving. Please refer to individual recipes and scale up or down depending on how many people you are cooking for.

WEEK FOUR MEAL PLANNER

 BREAKFAST

 LUNCH

DINNER

MONDAY
 TOTAL 776 CALS

Spiced Apple Overnight Oats (page 57)
256 calories

Creamy Cucumber & Smoked Salmon Open Sandwich (page 82)
108 calories

Spanish Chicken & Chorizo Stew (page 142)
412 calories

TUESDAY
 TOTAL 1342 CALS

Oat, Berry & Coconut Smoothie (page 58)
325 calories

Rainbow Vegetable & Feta Salad (page 96)
556 calories

Asian Salmon Burgers with Petits Pois & Potato Mash (page 148)
461 calories

WEDNESDAY
 TOTAL 952 CALS

Spinach & Egg French Toast (page 64)
312 calories

New Potato & Courgette Frittata (page 92)
225 calories

Shepherd's Pie with Veg Mash Topping (page 161)
415 calories

THURSDAY
 TOTAL 998 CALS

Egg, Bacon & Spinach Breakfast Muffins (page 70)
109 calories

Asian Chicken Salad (page 110)
487 calories

Zingy Courgette Carbonara (page 156)
402 calories

FRIDAY
 TOTAL 959 CALS

Green Smoothie (page 60)
151 calories

Filled Homemade Spinach Wraps (e.g. with vegetables and chicken) (page 88)
388 calories

Chicken Schnitzel with Three Veg Slaw (page 138)
420 calories

SATURDAY
 TOTAL 793 CALS

Egg, Bacon & Spinach Breakfast Muffins (page 70)
109 calories

Mediterranean Mackerel & Baked Rice (page 105)
388 calories

Five Vegetable Lasagne (page 129)
296 calories

SUNDAY
 TOTAL 779 CALS

Vegetable Fritters with Garlic Roast Tomatoes (page 74)
228 calories

Sunshine Soup (page 83)
129 calories

Pork Chops with Roast Vegetable Ratatouille (page 159)
422 calories

WEEK FOUR SHOPPING LIST

Fruit & Vegetables

1 banana

2 apples

3 lemons

3 limes

1 avocado

3 celery sticks

850g cherry tomatoes

1 cucumber

2 small cooked beetroot

1 bunch spring onions
   (plus an extra 2)

2 aubergines

1 bulb of fennel

1 butternut squash

15 carrots

8 courgettes

50g kale

300g mushrooms

350g new potatoes

700g potatoes

1 red cabbage

3 red peppers

100g sugar snap peas

1 swede

4 onions

3 red onions

3 heads of garlic

15g fresh basil

15g fresh chives

15g fresh coriander

10g fresh dill

30g fresh flat-leaf
   parsley

15g any soft fresh herbs

Dairy

55g unsalted butter

390g natural yoghurt

495ml semi-skimmed
   milk

20g Cheddar

100g feta

105g Parmesan

Meat & Fish

4 mackerel fillets

4 salmon fillets

75g smoked salmon

4 skinless, boneless
   chicken thighs

5 skinless, boneless
   chicken breasts

10 rashers unsmoked
   streaky bacon

4 pork chops (bone-in)

150g chorizo sausage

500g lean lamb mince

Frozen

175g frozen berries

590g frozen spinach

150g petits pois

**Store cupboard staples
(bread, eggs, dried
goods)**

10 slices bread

24 eggs

175g brown basmati rice

160g couscous

75g porridge oats

75g rice noodles

85g lasagne sheets

200g wholewheat
   spaghetti

1 × 400g tin chickpeas

1 × 400ml tin coconut
   milk

4 × 400g tins tinned
   tomatoes

100g panko
   breadcrumbs

180g black or green
   olives, pitted

200g jarred roasted
   peppers

Shopping list quantities reflect the number of people the recipe is stated as serving. Please refer to individual recipes and scale up or down depending on how many people you are cooking for.

INDEX

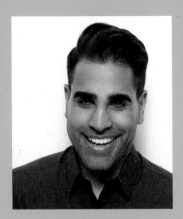

Dr Ranj Singh is an NHS clinician and one of the resident doctors on ITV's leading daytime series, *This Morning*. He is co-presenter of ITV's prime-time series *Save Money: Good Health*, and co-creating host of BAFTA-award-winning CBeebies series, *Get Well Soon*. Ranj was also a hugely popular contestant on 2018's *Strictly Come Dancing*. Off air, his work can be found in numerous magazines and websites, where he gives expert opinion and advice on a range of physical and mental health matters.

This book has been a labour of love for so many people and I can't thank each of them enough... but I'm going to have a go!

Firstly, thank you to everyone at Twofour for creating this fantastic show and letting me be a part of it. Never in my wildest dreams did I imagine that I would be co-presenting alongside Sian Williams, so I am incredibly grateful for this opportunity.

Thank you also to everyone at ITV for commissioning it, and especially to Shirley Patton for making this book possible.

A huge thanks has to go to the amazing team at Transworld: Michelle Signore, Becky Short, Emma Burton, Tom Chicken and Richard Ogle. Thanks for putting up with all my questions, queries and last-minute amendments. I couldn't ask for a better team to be behind my first proper book! Likewise thanks to everyone that has been instrumental in putting this book together, particularly Nicola Lafferty and Georgina Davies – without you I would be lost! Similarly, my gratitude goes out to Prof. Jane Smith, Emma and Alex Smith, Jo Roberts-Miller, Jamie Orlando Smith, Phil Mundy and Olivia Wardle.

However, the biggest thanks have to go to my wonderful team: my agent Craig Latto for not only always having my back but also being a great friend, KT Forster for being my literary rock and advocate, Jamie Brenner for being the best PA ever (even though he's not technically mine!), and Bryony Blake for the glam.

Last but by no means least, I want to express my heartfelt gratitude to all my friends and family for their endless love and support. I truly am the luckiest boy in the world. Without you I wouldn't have achieved a fraction of what I have done. To my parents especially: your hard work, sacrifice and support have made my dreams come true. I will be forever thankful and utterly proud of you.

This book is dedicated to Rohan, Sajjan and Olivia. May you grow up in a world that is loving, colourful and exciting. Chase your dreams and remember that anything is possible if you work hard enough.